Mechanical Ventilation in the Critically Ill Patient: International Nursing Perspectives

Editor

SANDRA GOLDSWORTHY

CRITICAL CARE NURSING CLINICS OF NORTH AMERICA

www.ccnursing.theclinics.com

Consulting Editor
JAN FOSTER

December 2016 • Volume 28 • Number 4

ELSEVIER

1600 John F. Kennedy Boulevard • Suite 1800 • Philadelphia, Pennsylvania, 19103-2899

http://www.theclinics.com

CRITICAL CARE NURSING CLINICS OF NORTH AMERICA Volume 28, Number 4
December 2016 ISSN 0899-5885, ISBN-13: 978-0-323-49626-1

Editor: Kerry Holland
Developmental Editor: Colleen Viola

Critical Care Nursing Clinics of North America (ISSN 0899-5885) is published quarterly by Elsevier Inc., 360 Park Avenue South, New York, NY 10010-1710. Months of issue are March, June, September, and December. Business and Editorial Offices: 1600 John F. Kennedy Blvd., Suite 1800, Philadelphia, PA 19103-2899. Periodicals postage paid at New York, NY and additional mailing offices. Subscription prices are $155.00 per year for US individuals, $370.00 per year for US institutions, $100.00 per year for US students and residents, $200.00 per year for Canadian individuals, $464.00 per year for Canadian institutions, $230.00 per year for international individuals, $464.00 per year for international institutions and $115.00 per year for Canadian and international students/residents. To receive student/resident rate, orders must be accompanied by name of affiliated institution, data of term, and the *signature* of program/residency coordinator on institution letterhead. Orders will be billed at individual rate until proof of status is received. Foreign air speed delivery is included in all *Clinics* subscription prices. All prices are subject to change without notice. **POSTMASTER:** Send address changes to *Critical Care Nursing Clinics of North America*, Elsevier Health Sciences Division, Subscription Customer Service, 3251 Riverport Lane, Maryland Heights, MO 63043. **Customer Service: 1-800-654-2452 (US and Canada); 314-447-8871 (outside US and Canada). Fax: 314-447-8029. E-mail:** JournalsCustomerService-usa@elsevier.com **(for print support) and** JournalsOnlineSupport-usa@elsevier.com **(for online support).**

Reprints. For copies of 100 or more of articles in this publication, please contact the Commercial Reprints Department, Elsevier Inc., 360 Park Avenue South, New York, New York, 10010-1710; Tel.: 212-633-3874, Fax: 212-633-3820, and E-mail: reprints@elsevier.com.

Critical Care Nursing Clinics of North America is covered in *MEDLINE/PubMed (Index Medicus), International Nursing Index, Nursing Citation Index, Cumulative Index to Nursing and Allied Health Literature, and RNdex Top 100.*

Contributors

CONSULTING EDITOR

JAN FOSTER, PhD, APRN, CNS
Formerly, Associate Professor, College of Nursing, Texas Woman's University, Houston; President, Nursing Inquiry and Intervention, Inc, The Woodlands, Texas

EDITOR

SANDRA GOLDSWORTHY, PhD, RN, CNCC(C), CMSN(C)
Associate Professor, Research Professorship in Simulation Education, Faculty of Nursing, University of Calgary, Calgary, Alberta, Canada

AUTHORS

THOMAS AHRENS, PhD, RN, FAAN
Research Scientist, Barnes-Jewish Hospital, St Louis, Missouri

SHAINDY ALEXANDER, BA, CCLS
Certified Child Life Specialist, Child Life Department, The Hospital for Sick Children, Toronto, Ontario, Canada

HEATHER BAID, RN, BSN, PGCHSCE, PGCert, MSc
Senior Lecturer and Intensive Care Pathway Leader, School of Health Sciences, University of Brighton, Brighton, United Kingdom

GLENN BARTON, MSN (Ed), RN
Curriculum/Instructional Designer, Department of Practice, Performance and Innovation, Health Systems Innovation and External Relations, Royal College of Physicians and Surgeons of Canada, Ottawa, Ontario, Canada

IRINA CHARANIA, RRT, BScH
Advanced Technical Skills Simulation Laboratory, University of Calgary, Calgary, Alberta, Canada

STACEY DALGLEISH, MN, NP
Neonatal Intensive Care Unit, Foothills Medical Centre, Calgary, Alberta, Canada

CATHY DANIELS, RN(EC), MS, NP-Paediatrics
Long-term Ventilation Program, Division of Respiratory Medicine, The Hospital for Sick Children, Toronto, Ontario, Canada

LEANNE DAVIDSON, HBSc, RRT
Clinician Educator, Respiratory Therapy, Cardiac Critical Care Unit, The Hospital for Sick Children, Toronto, Ontario, Canada

KAREN DRYDEN-PALMER, RN, MSN
Clinical Nurse Specialist, Paediatric Critical Care Unit, The Hospital for Sick Children, Toronto, Ontario, Canada

PAUL FULBROOK, RN, PhD, MSc, BSc(Hons), PGDipEduc
Director, Nursing Research and Practice Development Centre, The Prince Charles Hospital; Professor, School of Nursing, Midwifery and Paramedicine, Australian Catholic University, Brisbane, Australia

KITTY M. GARRETT, RN, MSN, CCRN, CCNS
Assistant Professor, Department of Physiological and Technological Nursing, College of Nursing, Augusta University, Augusta, Georgia

SANDRA GOLDSWORTHY, PhD, RN, CNCC(C), CMSN(C)
Associate Professor, Research Professorship in Simulation Education, Faculty of Nursing, University of Calgary, Calgary, Alberta, Canada

PAM HRUSKA, RN, MSc
Clinical Nurse Specialist, Adult Critical Care, Department of Critical Care Medicine, Alberta Health Services, Alberta, Canada

LINDA KOSTECKY, RN, BN
Neonatal Intensive Care Unit, Foothills Medical Centre, Calgary, Alberta, Canada

JASON MACARTNEY, RRT
Clinician Educator, Respiratory Therapy, Paediatric Critical Care Unit, Paediatric Intensive Care Unit, The Hospital for Sick Children, Toronto, Ontario, Canada

MAUREEN A. SECKEL, RN, APRN, MSN, ACNS-BC, CCNS, CCRN, FCCM
Medical Pulmonary Critical Care Clinical Nurse Specialist; Sepsis Coordinator, Christiana Care Health Services, Affiliated Faculty, College of Nursing, University of Delaware, Newark, Delaware

JACQUELINE SHEA, MScN, RN
Nurse Educator, Surgery, The Ottawa Hospital, General Campus, Ottawa, Ontario, Canada

FAIZA SYED, BHSC, RRT
Long-term Ventilation Program, Division of Respiratory Medicine, The Hospital for Sick Children, Toronto, Ontario, Canada

BRANDI VANDERSPANK-WRIGHT, PhD, RN, CNCC(C)
Assistant Professor, Faculty of Health Sciences, School of Nursing, University of Ottawa, Ottawa, Ontario, Canada

DARIAN WARD, RN, MN, BN, PGCertCritCare, PGDipProfStud
Director of Education, Training and Research, Wide Bay Hospital and Health Service, Queensland, Australia

Contents

A foundational skill for critical care nurses caring for mechanically ventilated patients. This paper describes challenges and opportunities in preparing nurses to transition into the intensive care environment. Hospitals invest significant funding in educational programs for new critical care nurses so that they can transition effectively into the critical care environment. Simulation has been shown to impact self-efficacy and performance. This paper describes the integration of mechanical ventilation education into a case-based simulation program and the results of a study measuring self-efficacy and transfer of learning before and after the implementation of a simulation intervention.

Critically ill patients requiring mechanical ventilation are least likely to be mobilized and, as a result, are at-risk for prolonged complications from weakness. The use of bed rest and sedation when caring for mechanically ventilated patients is likely shaped by historical practice; however, this review demonstrates early mobilization, with little to no sedation, is possible and safe. Assessing readiness for mobilization in context of progressing patients from passive to active activities can lead to long-term benefits and has been achievable with resource-efficient implementations and team work.

Critical care nurses constitute front-line care provision for patients in the intensive care unit (ICU). Hypoxemic respiratory compromise/failure is a primary reason that patients require ICU admission and mechanical ventilation. Critical care nurses must possess advanced knowledge, skill, and judgment when caring for these patients to ensure that interventions aimed at optimizing oxygenation are both effective and safe. This article discusses fundamental aspects of respiratory physiology and clinical indices used to describe oxygenation status. Key nursing interventions including patient assessment, positioning, pharmacology, and managing hemodynamic parameters are discussed, emphasizing their effects toward mitigating ventilation–perfusion mismatch and optimizing oxygenation.

Nursing management of pain, agitation, and delirium in mechanically ventilated patients is a challenge in critical care. Oversedation can lead to delayed extubation, prolonged ventilator days, unnecessary neurologic testing, and complications such as weakness and delirium. Undersedation can lead to self-extubation, invasive line removal, unnecessary patient distress, and injury to self or others. Acquiring an optimal level of sedation requires the bedside nurse to be more vigilant than ever with patient assessment and medication titration. This article provides a historical perspective of the management of pain, agitation, and delirium, and disseminates information contained in revised Society for Critical Care Medicine Clinical Practice Guidelines (January 2013) to promote their implementation in day-to-day nursing care.

Mechanical ventilation is a fundamental aspect of critical care practice to help meet the respiratory needs of critically ill patients. Complications can occur though, as a direct result of being mechanically ventilated, or indirectly because of a secondary process. Preventing, identifying, and managing these complications significantly contribute to the role and responsibilities of critical care nurses in promoting patient safety. This article reviews common ventilator-associated events, including both infectious (eg, ventilator-associated pneumonia) and noninfectious causes (eg, acute respiratory distress syndrome, pulmonary edema, pleural effusion, and atelectasis).

Mechanical ventilation is often required to support the recovery of critically ill children. Critical care nurses must understand the unique needs of the children and design supportive care that is sensitive to their changing physiology, developmental stage, and socioemotional needs. This article describes the unique considerations in providing care for mechanically ventilated children. It addresses invasive and noninvasive ventilation and the needs of long-term ventilated children and family in critical care. Supportive nursing care that is aligned with the unique needs of the critically ill child is paramount to ensuring best outcomes for these vulnerable patients.

Care of infants supported with mechanical ventilation is complex, time intensive, and requires constant vigilance by an expertly prepared health care team. Current evidence must guide nursing practice regarding ventilated neonates. This article highlights the importance of common language to establish a shared mental model and enhance clear communication among the interprofessional team. Knowledge regarding the underpinnings of an open lung strategy and the interplay between the pathophysiology and individual infant's response to a specific ventilator strategy is most likely to result in a positive clinical outcome.

The risks imposed by mechanical ventilation can be mitigated by nurses' use of strategies that promote early but appropriate reduction of ventilatory support and timely extubation. Weaning from mechanical ventilation is confounded by the multiple impacts of critical illness on the body's systems. Effective weaning strategies that combine several interventions that optimize weaning readiness and assess readiness to wean, and use a weaning protocol in association with spontaneous breathing trials, are likely to reduce the requirement for mechanical ventilatory support in a timely manner. Weaning strategies should be reviewed and updated regularly to ensure congruence with the best available evidence.

Special Article

There are two important recent changes in sepsis care. The first key change is the 2016 Sepsis-3 definitions from the recent consensus workgroup with new sepsis and septic shock definitions. Useful tools for assessing patients that have a greater risk of mortality include Sequential Organ Failure Assessment (SOFA) in intensive care units and quick SOFA outside intensive care units. The second change involves management of fluid resuscitation and measures of volume responsiveness. Measures such as blood pressure and central venous pressure are not reliable. Fluid challenges and responsiveness should be based on stroke volume change of greater than 10%.

CRITICAL CARE NURSING
CLINICS OF NORTH AMERICA

THE CLINICS ARE AVAILABLE ONLINE!
Access your subscription at:
www.theclinics.com

Preface

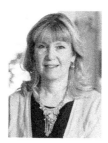

Sandra Goldsworthy, PhD, RN, CNCC(C), CMSN(C)
Editor

In this special issue of *Critical Care Nursing Clinics of North America*, care of the mechanically ventilated patient in critical care is explored. These articles have been written by critical care nurse experts and their teams and provide a broad range of topics in this area of specialty. The authors of these articles represent a diverse geographical area, including Canada, Australia, Britain, and the United States.

Care of the mechanically ventilated patient in the intensive care unit (ICU) is a foundational competency. Ongoing professional development in this area allows critical care nurses and critical care teams to continue to stay on the leading edge of evidence-informed practice in this area. We hope that you will find many practical applications from the articles presented in this issue that you can apply in your everyday practice.

Composition of critical care teams varies globally, with respiratory therapists being unique to North America. Critical care nurses collaborate with a variety of health professionals in the ICU and need to be vigilant in maintaining their skill in caring for the critically ill mechanically ventilated patient. Mechanical ventilation has been listed as one of the ICU competencies novice nurses in ICU feel least confident about.

In this issue, topics such as optimizing oxygenation and preventing complications of mechanical ventilation are discussed. Special situation articles have also been added that discuss mechanical ventilation in the pediatric and neonatal patient. Innovative simulation educational strategies for nurses transitioning into ICU are also presented.

We hope you find these articles that were written by nurses for nurses to be practical, useful, and relevant in your bedside practice in the ICU.

Sandra Goldsworthy, PhD, RN, CNCC(C), CMSN(C)
Associate Professor
Research Professorship in Simulation Education
Faculty of Nursing
University of Calgary
2500 University Drive Northwest
Calgary, Alberta T2N 1N4, Canada

E-mail address:
Sandra.goldsworthy@ucalgary.ca

Crit Care Nurs Clin N Am 28 (2016) ix
http://dx.doi.org/10.1016/j.cnc.2016.09.013
0899-5885/16/© 2016 Published by Elsevier Inc.

ccnursing.theclinics.com

Mechanical Ventilation Education and Transition of Critical Care Nurses into Practice

Sandra Goldsworthy, PhD, RN, CNCC(C), CMSN(C)

KEYWORDS

- Critical care • Mechanical ventilation • Nurse • Simulation • Education
- Self-efficacy • Transfer of learning

KEY POINTS

- A new tool for measuring critical care self-efficacy was developed for this study.
- A nurses' level of self-efficacy in approaching a new skills has been shown to impact their ability to transfer learning from the educational setting to the practice setting.
- High-fidelity simulation mimics the practice setting and allows students to practice in a safe setting where the repetition and reflective debriefing occur to deepen and extend their learning.
- Novice critical care nurses listed mechanical ventilation as one of the critical care competencies about which they felt least confident.

INTRODUCTION

Critical care nurses are required to have specialized skills and knowledge to enable them to critically think rapidly in life and death situations. High-level cognitive and emotional competencies are associated with the technical and relational dilemmas encountered daily in these settings. One of the specific skill sets that is foundational for critical care nurses is to be able to competently care for mechanically ventilated patients. This paper describes the unique challenges and opportunities in preparing nurses to transition into the intensive care environment in relation to mechanical ventilation. Results of a longitudinal quasiexperimental study among critical care nurses is described and the relationship among critical care self-efficacy, general self-efficacy (GSE), and transfer of learning (TOL) is explored. Furthermore, the simulation intervention used as a teaching/learning strategy in this study is discussed.

Faculty of Nursing, University of Calgary, 2500 University Drive Northwest, Calgary, Alberta T2N 1N4, Canada
E-mail address: Sandra.goldsworthy@ucalgary.ca

Crit Care Nurs Clin N Am 28 (2016) 399–412
http://dx.doi.org/10.1016/j.cnc.2016.07.001
0899-5885/16/© 2016 Elsevier Inc. All rights reserved.

SELF-EFFICACY

Self-efficacy plays an important role in moderating TOL.[1] It has been shown to moderate the relationship between training and newcomer adjustment.[2] When new employees do not adjust well in the initial phase of a job, it can lead to disengagement and turnover. Self-efficacy has also been shown to be strongly related to work performance and can be developed through mastery experiences, which largely involve 'hands-on' learning.[3] The opportunity to repeat tasks, such as simulated learning experiences, is related to increased levels of self-efficacy or the belief that one can perform the task.

An individual's self-efficacy can influence how they approach tasks and new challenges, such as learning situations. Self-efficacy is conceptualized as being general or domain specific. GSE is a traitlike generality dimension defined as "an individual's perception of their ability to perform across a variety of situations."[4] Domain-specific self-efficacy refers to how an individual feels capable of approaching and performing specific tasks, such as competencies in critical care.[4] Self-efficacy is differentiated conceptually from similar constructs, like self-esteem, which is considered to be a relatively stable 'trait.' Situational self-efficacy, in contrast, is considered to be a 'state' that is dynamic in time and in different contexts.[5] The concept of self-efficacy arises from social cognitive theory, in which an individual's reactions and actions are based on what the individual has observed in others.[4] Self-efficacy is broadly defined as "people's judgements about their capabilities to organize and execute courses of action required to attain designated types of performance; it is concerned not with the skills one has but with judgments of what one can do with whatever skills one possesses."[4]

Domain-specific self-efficacy is typically developed through mastery experiences and vicarious learning and modeling by observing others perform the task.[4] Mastery experiences are largely gained through hands-on experience, such as through practice in the clinical setting with patients or through practice in the simulation laboratory with simulated patients. Bandura[3] (1986) also argued that self-efficacy develops with the opportunity to repeat tasks. Individuals who have increased levels of self-efficacy feel they can have an impact on their environment, whereas individuals with low levels of self-efficacy view problems as unmanageable and insurmountable. Individuals with low self-efficacy may avoid a situation, instead of facing a task, if they feel that they may not be able to do it.

Research on self-efficacy in relation to training interventions is important in the understanding of effective training. An individual with greater self-efficacy is more likely to make an effort and persist longer at a task, compared with those with lesser self-efficacy. Self-efficacy has been shown to significantly influence academic success, persistence, and career competency (Bandura, 1993).[6] Task-specific self-efficacy has also been shown to influence a novice's adjustment to the workplace.[2,7] Furthermore, domain-specific self-efficacy has been operationalized in the literature as a moderator of training methods for posttraining self-efficacy and performance.[8]

Self-efficacy can be enhanced through formal training programs, especially when the individual perceives the training to be similar to the work environment where they will be applying their skills.[8] Tannenbaum and colleagues[9] had similar findings: when training meets the participant's expectations, their organizational commitment, self-efficacy, and training motivation are influenced positively. Self-efficacy has also been found to moderate training methods for outcomes such as TOL[2,10] and has been found to be a key variable in TOL research.[11] TOL refers to the ability to transfer skills learned in the educational environment (ie, the simulation laboratory) to the practice area. Colquitt and colleagues[12] demonstrated that self-efficacy predicts motivation to learn. Individuals with increased levels of self-efficacy will have a greater likelihood of persevering and performing on the job. In summary, self-efficacy is a motivational construct that influences whether or not an individual believes they can complete the task, which influences their effort, coping, and persistence.

Studies in the nursing population have explored the influence of self-efficacy and performance for specific tasks. In 1 study exploring self-efficacy in the nursing population, a simulation intervention was delivered to 112 undergraduate nursing students.[13] In the intervention, the training included maternal–child scenarios that mimicked the real practice settings, which were delivered via high-fidelity patient simulators. The results showed a significant increase in the levels of self-efficacy when pretests were compared with the posttest measures.[13]

Similar results were found in a US study of 49 registered nurses where high-fidelity simulation training was conducted for the management of preeclampsia and eclampsia. Nurse levels of self-efficacy were significantly increased when the pretests and posttests were compared.[14] In addition, the levels of self-efficacy were found to be sustained over time when the posttests were readministered at 8 weeks after the intervention. In this single group design, the nurses also reported being highly satisfied with simulation as an effective teaching strategy.

Chen and colleagues[15] (2008) found that "high general self-efficacy can maintain employees' work motivation throughout rapidly changing stressful job demands and circumstances and buffer them from the potentially demotivating impact of failure." In the few studies dealing with simulation and self-efficacy, high-fidelity simulation has been shown to be positively related to both GSE and situation-specific self-efficacy among nurses.

TRANSFER OF LEARNING

Organizations are not only interested in retaining nurses, but in retaining employees who are high performers and able to successfully transfer learning into the practice environment. Every year, hospitals invest a significant amount of funding into educational programs to provide the necessary training for nurses who are new to critical care, so that they can transition effectively into the critical care environment. The programs are designed to enhance knowledge, competency, and judgment for providing safe patient care to critically ill patients. Many of the competencies learned in these programs are related to high-risk skills, such as care of the mechanically ventilated patient that must be performed often in rapidly changing patient conditions. Traditional orientations for critical care nurses include a theoretic component and a preceptored clinical component. Ideally, organizations would like to have maximal return on their investment for the programs to ensure that the training is effective for the transfer of skills and competencies into practice.

TOL refers to a change in behavior on the job once training has been received.[16] Positive TOL is used interchangeably in the literature with transfer of training, which is defined as the degree to which trainees effectively apply knowledge, skills, and attitudes gained in the training context to the job[17] and the extent to which the learning that results from the training experience transfers to the job and leads to meaningful changes in work performance.[18] The most frequently cited TOL model is the Baldwin and Ford (1988) model.[19] This framework includes 3 main components: training inputs (trainee characteristics, training design, and work environment factors), training outputs (acquisition of knowledge and skills during training), and conditions of transfer (generalization of knowledge and skills and the maintenance of skills learned over time). Trainee characteristics include self-efficacy and motivation, and the training design includes method of training and use of training objectives. In addition, specific work environment characteristics include transfer climate, peer and supervisor support, and opportunities or barriers to applying the learned behaviors in the work setting.

Learners who are motivated are more likely to engage in learning.[20] Examples of factors that promote transfer include supervisor and peer encouragement to use new skills, task cues that remind employee to use new skills, and rewards for using new skills in a work setting. Organizations that encourage and promote continuous learning have systems in place for sharing knowledge and learning is rewarded and supported by managers. In contrast, some obstacles in the work environment have been shown to inhibit transfer,[16] for example, work conditions (time pressures, few opportunities to use skills, and inadequate equipment), lack of peer support, and lack of management support.

Two of the major metaanalyses in the area of TOL were conducted by Arthur and colleagues[21] and by Blume and colleagues.[22] The focus of the metaanalysis by Arthur and associates was measurement of effectiveness of training in organizations specifically related to design and evaluation features. Most studies with effective training were found to use multiple training methods (ie, lecture and psychomotor skill application). The results showed that, for maximal training effectiveness, the skills required in the workplace must be matched with the training and evaluation method. For example, in the nursing training context, high-fidelity human simulators must be used to create a realistic clinical environment in the laboratory so that nurses can learn specific skills and competencies.

The second major metaanalysis, by Blume and colleagues,[22] included 89 studies and explored the predictive factors of transfer of training. The primary predictors that were highlighted in the metaanalysis were trainee characteristics, work environment characteristics, and the training intervention. For the 3 categories, the research was focused mainly on the training design and delivery methods. Transfer climate was found to have the strongest relationship with TOL.

A large systematic review and metaanalysis was conducted to examine technology-enhanced simulation used in health professions education.[23] In the metaanalysis, 609 eligible studies were found, and of these, 137 were randomized studies and 405 used a single group pretest–posttest design. The results showed a small to moderate effect that favored simulation in comparison with other instructional strategies (ie, video, lecture, and small group). Nurses and nursing students accounted for 79 of the studies that were reviewed. This analysis extracted studies that involved a broad spectrum of simulation, across all fidelity levels of simulators and other simulation strategies, including the use of cadavers.

In one of the few studies on performance improvement in the clinical setting, the effect of a simulation activity was examined on the performance of established interprofessional critical care unit teams. The sample included 40 teams composed of 1 doctor and 3 nurses from 9 different critical care units in 8 hospitals in New Zealand.[24] Teams participated in cardiac and airway scenarios and the results of the 10-hour intervention showed an improvement in team work and evidence for changes to patient management. In another simulation intervention study of 38 medical–surgical registered nurses in Australia, simulation was shown to have positive effects on performance. The intervention consisted of 14 hours of theory related to clinical emergencies that could lead to cardiac arrest. The lecture was followed by 3 hours of practice in the simulation laboratory with high-fidelity simulators. The results showed that nurses' confidence and perceived technical and nontechnical skills in responding to patient emergencies were enhanced after simulation.[25] To promote TOL, employees require specific conditions in the immediate work environment that promote TOL, such as manager support, adequacy of resources, and opportunity to practice skills.

SIMULATION

Although nurses have indicated they value professional development opportunities at all career stages, no research has examined which method of educational delivery is the most effective in retaining nurses. An educational strategy that has been gaining traction within nursing over the last 5 to 10 years is the use of high-fidelity human simulators.[26] High-fidelity simulation mimics the practice setting and allows students to practice in a safe setting where the repetition of skills can occur along with reflective debriefing to deepen and possibly extend the learning that occurs during the simulation. A recent systematic review evaluated the use of simulation in undergraduate education. In the 101 research papers that were examined, 7 themes emerged from the synthesis of the research.[27] The themes included confidence/self-efficacy, satisfaction, skills/knowledge, and anxiety/stress. The researchers concluded that more robust simulation research is needed in nursing. In another recent systematic review that examined simulation-based learning in nursing education, a total of 12 studies were included in the final review.[28] The authors found that simulation improved knowledge/skill, critical thinking, and confidence among nurses. The research also showed that simulation may be advantageous over other teaching methods, depending on the context, method, and whether or not simulation best practices were followed. Examples of best practices in simulation include curriculum-based scenarios, use of a 3-step simulation process (briefing, simulation, and debriefing), and preparation of the physical environment that closely mimics the practice setting.[29]

A few studies have explored the impact of skills learned in simulation and how this transfers to the practice setting. In a US study of critical care nurses (n = 24, >880 medication doses) that compared a simulation intervention versus traditional lecture, and the influence on medication error rates in critically ill patients, significantly fewer medication errors occurred in the group that received the simulation intervention.[30] Another US study compared lecture with simulation among senior-level nursing students (n = 54) and found that neither teaching strategy was effective in isolation.[31]

A small number of research studies on simulation have demonstrated an increased clinical performance and self-efficacy in specific situations, such as among nursing students (n = 54) in caring for patients with distributive shock,[31] registered nurses (n = 47) handling obstetric emergencies such as eclampsia and preeclampsia,[14] preparing nursing students (n = 120) for pediatric practice settings,[32] and decreasing medication administration errors among nursing students (n = 54) in acute medical surgical practice settings.[33]

SUMMARY OF THE LITERATURE

A nurses' level of self-efficacy in approaching a new skills has been shown to impact their ability to transfer learning from the educational setting (ie, simulation laboratory) to the practice setting. Simulation as a teaching/learning strategy allows individuals to practice new high-risk skills in a safe environment while at the same time positively impacting performance and self-efficacy. Lack of confidence in performing skills such as caring for a mechanically ventilated critically ill patient can impact performance and adjustment as new nurses' transition into the intensive care unit (ICU). In the next section, results of a study that explored the impact of an educational intervention that included simulation and was aimed at transition of new nurses into ICU.[34] The intervention included simulation cases designed to prepare the nurse to care for mechanically ventilated patients.

METHOD

This study used a quasiexperimental design to primarily test the effects of a professional development intervention on critical care nurses' intent to stay. In addition, the relationship between GSE, critical care self-efficacy, and TOL was explored.

Sample

Participants included a convenience sample of critical care nurses from hospitals in central Canada who had attended a professional development program that consisted of simulation and practicum components, and a comparison group that consisted of a random sample of Canadian critical care nurses obtained from the professional licensure registry in the same province (n = 363).

Measures

The measures used in this study included GSE, critical care self-efficacy, and TOL. All study measures showed good internal consistency with alpha coefficients of greater than 0.79 critical care self-efficacy (α = .85 treatment group and α = .91, comparison group): GSE, 0.79 treatment and 0.88 control; TOL, 0.84 treatment only. The TOL Scale was adapted to the critical care nursing context from the Facteau and colleagues'[34] 9-item measure. The adapted measure contains 6 items and is measured on a 5-point response scale ranging from 1 (strongly disagree) to 5 (strongly agree) that assesses how well the individual perceives that they have transferred the learning from the intervention into the critical care practice setting.[35] Domain-specific self-efficacy was measured by the Critical Care Nursing Self-efficacy Scale that was researcher developed using Bandura's guide for developing domain specific self-efficacy scales, with reference to 10 core critical care nursing competencies that included hemodynamic monitoring, arrhythmia interpretation, 12-lead electrocardiograph interpretation, vasoactive drip calculation, mechanical ventilation, recognition of hemodynamic instability, and ability to prioritize in rapidly changing situations. This 10-item scale is measured on a scale of 0 to 100 points that yields a final composite score of 0 to 1000. The Cronbach's alpha for the researcher developed Critical Care Self-efficacy Scale was 0.83.

In addition to the measurement of domain specific critical care self-efficacy, a GSE measure was used as a baseline in the initial survey to all participants. The GSE measure used was the 10-item Jerusalem and Schwartzer scale[36,37] The measure is unidimensional and is scored on a Likert scale of 1 to 4 (from 1 [hardly true] to 4 [exactly true]) when the sum is calculated a final composite score ranging from 10 to 40 is produced.

Professional Development Intervention

The professional development intervention was a 324-hour self-paced critical care certificate program offered over a maximum of a 1-year period. The program included the following 3 components: (a) 6 instructor-facilitated online learning modules offered in an asynchronous format, (b) an onsite instructor-facilitated 39-hour high fidelity simulation course held over 2 weekends, and (c) a preceptored practicum over ten 12-hour shifts in an adult critical care unit. This professional development intervention is intended to prepare registered nurses for the critical care practice setting. The program curriculum is standardized and has been delivered for 5 years with a consistent faculty team. Traditional models of critical care training for nurses entering critical care include a condensed classroom format to deliver theory followed by a practicum course. This program was unique compared with traditional critical care training models, because it is composed of 3 discrete training modalities, with a distinct sequencing model of interactive online learning followed by an intensive simulation laboratory course and finally a practicum component.

The Simulation Intervention Component

Before the simulation component, all nurse participants had successfully completed 6 online theory courses. The 6 online courses included an introduction to online learning, and 5 critical care theory courses focusing on the following topic areas: advanced pathophysiology, cardiac, respiratory, neurologic, and gastrointestinal/endocrine/renal. The respiratory course included foundational topics related to care of the mechanically ventilated patient, such as oxygen therapy, arterial blood gas analysis, mechanical ventilation modes, nursing management at the bedside, weaning, and pharmacology related to mechanical ventilation.[38] The simulation component of the intervention included 39 hours of simulated critical care cases conducted within the simulation laboratory. Participation in the cases included 3 preparation stations that included arrhythmia/12-lead electrocardiograph interpretation, management of mechanical ventilation and hemodynamic monitoring management (ie, arterial lines and pulmonary artery catheters). After completing the preparation stations, each student participated in 9 critical care cases that consisted of patients experiencing respiratory distress/acute respiratory failure, septic shock, hypovolemic shock, myocardial infarction, abdominal aortic aneurysm repair, hemodynamic instability, end-of-life care (mock family conference), acute renal failure, and head injury/trauma (**Fig. 1**).

Each case was delivered via a predetermined template that included learning objectives, pretest questions, an initial patient phase, an evolving patient phase, and a conclusion phase. The case was followed by guided debriefing and posttest questions. The duration of each case was 60 minutes and included 10 minutes for prebrief and review of the learning objectives, a 20-minute case, and 30 minutes for debriefing and a postintervention quiz.

All 8 instructors were registered nurses with more than 25 years each of critical care practice experience. Each of the instructors had mentored with the core critical care simulation team before independently running simulation cases. The evaluation and testing of the students was completed by instructors via competency-based checklists that were created by a team of critical care experts and had been trialed over a 5-year period before being used in the study.

Mechanical Ventilation Education Integration

Mechanical ventilation was integrated into case-based simulations and followed international best practices for simulation.[30] Specifically, the cases including mechanical ventilation learning followed a 3 pronged approach of prebriefing, simulation activity, and debriefing. Prebriefing is designed to provide an orientation and a context to the case by preparing students through a series of activities (**Table 1**). Initially, students completed an 8-month online theory component that included the care of mechanically ventilated patient. Indications for ventilation, nursing care, complications, modes, and trouble-shooting alarms were among the topics covered in the online course.[38]

Once the nurses arrived for the 2 weekends of simulation (39 hours in total), they were assigned specific roles and worked in groups of 3 to 5 to care for the "patient."

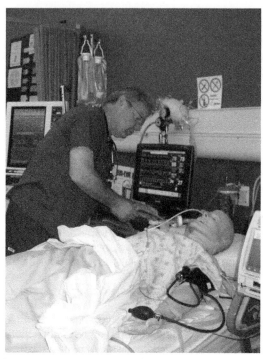

Fig. 1. Simulation laboratory.

The approach to teaching care of the mechanically ventilated patient incorporated a scaffolding approach designed to build confidence and competence through starting with less complex skills and cases (ie, acute respiratory distress case, mechanical ventilation skill station focusing on trouble-shooting alarms and arterial blood gas review) and progressing to more complex, or major cases such as acute respiratory distress syndrome (**Fig. 2**).[34]

All participants had an opportunity to repeat the cases on the second weekend. During each simulation major case, participants were evaluated based on specific competency checklists that had been developed previously by a team of critical care nurse experts and validated (**Table 2**). Once the simulation was complete each small group participated in a debriefing of the simulation.

Table 1	
Examples of ARDS pretest questions (before simulation) and posttest questions (after simulation)	
ARDS Pretest Questions (Administered Before the Simulation)	**ARDS Posttest Questions (Administered After the Simulation)**
1. Discuss potential causes of ARDS.	1. Describe types of pharmacologic interventions that may be used as supportive treatment in ARDS.
2. What is the main goal in treatment of ARDS?	2. What interventions can help prevent complications in ARDS?

Abbreviation: ARDS, acute respiratory distress syndrome.

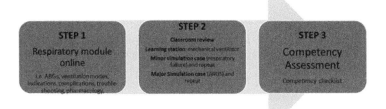

Fig. 2. Integration of mechanical ventilation competencies: pedagogical approach. ABGs, arterial blood gases.

Table 2
Mechanical ventilation competency checklist example: excerpted from ARDS simulation case

Competency	Examples	Met	Unmet	Comments
1. Demonstrates ability to correctly interpret arrhythmia.	Uses a systematic approach for non–life-threatening arrhythmias. Calls for assistance as needed.			
2. Demonstrates safe management of oxygenation.	Can differentiate between ventilation modes, indications, and contraindications. Troubleshoots ventilator alarms. Recognizes and responds to below normal oxygen saturation levels. Calls for assistance as needed.			
3. Demonstrates ability to quickly identify and respond to a patient's rapidly deteriorating condition.	Recognizes and responds to abnormal assessments and critical findings (ie, ++ secretions, crackles, respiratory distress, hyper or hypoventilation, patient/ ventilator asynchrony, deteriorating level of consciousness and increased work of breathing).			
4. Troubleshoots mechanical ventilator alarms anticipates ventilator changes based on ABGs and patient's changing condition.	Accurately interprets laboratory values. Suctions ETT as appropriate based on assessment. Accurately assesses and records any changes in patient status.			
5. Demonstrates safe administration of pharmacologic agents.	Dopamine infusion. Sedation administration.			
Feedback:				
Instructor name:				

Abbreviations: ARDS, acute respiratory distress syndrome; ETT, endotracheal tube.

RESULTS

The study found that critical care self-efficacy (ie, one's confidence in approaching critical care competencies) correlated positively with GSE (confidence in approaching new tasks in general; $r = 0.24$). In addition, critical care self-efficacy positively correlated with TOL (ie, the ability to transfer learned skills into the ICU; $r = 0.26$). Furthermore, GSE also was positively correlated with TOL ($r = 0.36$) critical care self-efficacy, positively correlated with TOL ($r = 0.26$), and TOL and GSE positively correlated ($r = 0.36$).

Among nurses receiving the simulation intervention (novice ICU nurses), the top 3 competencies that nurses rated as feeling the most confident in performing were arterial blood gas interpretation, arterial line management, and prioritization of a critical care patient. The critical care competencies the nurses receiving the simulation intervention rated as their least confident in performing were wedging a pulmonary artery catheter, performing a cardiac output, and mechanical ventilation. In contrast, the experienced nurse group (comparison group) that did not receive the simulation intervention said they felt most confident in arterial line management, arrhythmia interpretation, and mechanical ventilation and least confident in performing cardiac outputs, wedging a pulmonary artery catheter, and interpreting 12-lead electrocardiographs (**Box 1**).

IMPLICATIONS FOR NURSING EDUCATION

Nurses transitioning into a critical care specialty area typically require additional preparation beyond the undergraduate level to acquire the competencies required to safely practice in the ICU. Historically, critical care programs to prepare nurses for critical care have been composed of a classroom theoretical component followed by a preceptored practicum. In this study, the critical care program consisted of 3 discrete components: online, simulation, and a preceptored practicum.

A new critical care self-efficacy tool was created for this research and provides an opportunity to evaluate which competencies critical care nurses feel least confident about performing. Simulation training allows nurses to be evaluated before proceeding to the practice setting and provides an assessment on where additional training may be required.

Box 1
Critical care self-efficacy competency variables

- Arrhythmia interpretation
- Interpretation of a 12-lead electrocardiograph
- Mechanical ventilation
- Arterial blood gas interpretation
- Managing a cardiac arrest
- Performing a cardiac output
- Wedging a pulmonary artery catheter
- Prioritizing care for a critically ill patient
- Calculation of vasoactive infusion dosages
- Managing an arterial line

The results of this study suggest that professional development that includes simulation may be an effective strategy for increasing confidence and allows the nurse to practice in a 'safe' environment where no harm will occur to a patient while the nurse is learning new high-risk competencies. These findings have implications for nurse educators in the creation and provision of effective training programs for nurses transitioning to critical care and also for existing staff in ICU. In planning professional development opportunities, nurse educators need to give attention to competencies nurses report they are the least confident in and consider designing orientations and critical care programs that will enhance practice opportunities by providing intensive case based simulation scenarios. Simulation provides opportunity for practice with skills not frequently seen in the ICU (high-risk/low-frequency skills). The findings suggest that attention needs to be given to the ongoing learning needs of not only nurses new to critical care, but also to experienced ICU nurse and consideration given to professional development opportunities in this group as well. Other implications for nurse educators include the notion of creating an environment conducive to TOL. Creating a positive transfer climate includes factors, such as opportunity to practice and apply new skills, manager and peer support, encouragement, and adequate resources.

The findings in this study suggest that professional development opportunities should be provided to all ICU nurses on an ongoing basis and that consideration to the most effective educational strategy (ie, simulation) is made before program delivery. This study provided new knowledge in the area of critical care self-efficacy among ICU nurses and further study is needed in developing additional competencies for testing, such as communication-based competencies that could include family, patients, and other health care team members. In addition, further study is needed to examine the period immediately after the preceptorship period ends; the findings in this study showed that critical care self-efficacy means decreased slightly at the end of the practicum phase of the intervention, which coincides approximately with the end of the preceptorship period of the orientation. More exploration of nurses' self-efficacy is needed further into their tenure in ICU to determine whether critical care self-efficacy levels begin to increase again as the nurse adjusts to the critical care practice setting.

Specifically, future research is needed to determine which educational strategies are the most effective in retaining nurses and facilitating adjustment during initial tenure in the ICU. Newer emerging simulation technologies for teaching and learning, such as virtual simulation or a hybrid approach of combining high-fidelity simulation and virtual simulation, could be explored in relation to which method is the most effective at increasing self-efficacy and the ability to transfer or apply the learning into the practice setting.

SUMMARY

Hospitals make large financial investments to provide orientation programs to assist nurses in transitioning into the critical care setting. To determine whether or not the organization is receiving a good return on its investment, the idea of TOL is being used to measure organizational and workplace outcomes, such as performance. Hospitals are also interested in whether or not employees can apply the skills they learn in training to the practice setting, to provide safe, high-quality care. Unhealthy work environments that lack manager support and have inadequate resources are seen as having obstacles in the TOL to employees. TOL increases when the training environment is similar to the practice setting and when employees have opportunities to practice their skills immediately after training. Simulation provides the opportunity to create realistic settings for learning, such skills as caring for the mechanically ventilated patients. Simulation has been shown to be superior to other educational methods in improving performance and transfer/application of learning in the practice setting.[23,28]

Simulation has emerged in recent years as an educational strategy for nurses and has been shown to increase levels of self-efficacy, competence, and performance. Further research is needed in this area to establish the influences of simulation and the TOL (ie, for skills such as caring for the mechanically ventilated patient) to the practice setting. Much of the simulation research has been conducted in simulation labs without considering the transfers of learning behaviors over time.

REFERENCES

1. Gist M, Stevens C, Bavetta A. Effects of a self-efficacy post training intervention on the acquisition of complex interpersonal skills. Person Psychol 1991;44: 837–61.
2. Saks A. Longitudinal field investigation of moderating and mediating effects of self-efficacy on the relationship between training and newcomer adjustment. J Appl Psychol 1995;80:211–25.
3. Bandura A. Social foundations of thought and action: a social-cognitive view. Englewood Cliffs (NJ): Prentice Hall; 1986.
4. Judge T, Erez A, Bono J. The power of being positive: the relation between positive self-concept and job performance. Hum Perform 1998;11(2/3):167–87.
5. Gist M, Mitchell T. Self-efficacy: a theoretical analysis of its determinants and malleability. Acad Manage Rev 1992;17(2):183–211.
6. Bandura A. Perceived self-efficacy in cognitive development and functioning. Educ Psychol 1993;28(2):117–48.
7. Stajkovic A, Luthans F. Self-efficacy and work related performance: a meta-analysis. Psychol Bull 1998;124(2):240–61.
8. Louthans F, Youssef C. Emerging positive organizational behaviour. J Manag 2007;33(3):321–49.
9. Tannenbaum S, Mathieu J, Salas E, et al. Meeting trainees expectations: the influence of training fulfillment on the development of commitment, self-efficacy and motivation. J Appl Psychol 1991;76(6):759–69.
10. Pham N, Mien S, Gijselaers W. Understanding training transfer effects from a motivational perspective: a test for MBA programmes. Business Leadership Review. 2010.
11. Machin M, Fogarty G. The effects of self-efficacy, motivation to transfer and situational constraints on transfer intentions and transfer of training. Perform Improv Q 1997;10(2):98–115.
12. Colquitt J, Lepine J, Noe R. Toward an integrative theory of training and motivation: a meta-analysis of 20 years of research. J Appl Psychol 2000;85(5):678–707.
13. Bambini D, Washburn J, Perkins R. Outcomes of clinical simulation for novice nursing students: communication, confidence, clinical judgment. Nurs Educ Perspect 2009;30(2):79–82.
14. Christian A, Krumwiede N. Simulation enhances self-efficacy in the management of preeclampsia and eclampsia in obstetrical staff nurses. Clin Simul Nurs 2013; 9(9):e369–77.
15. Chen H, Chu C, Wang Y, et al. Turnover factors revisited: a longitudinal study of Taiwan-based staff nurses. Int J Nurs Stud 2008;45:277–85.

16. Noe R. Employee training and development. 4th edition. Boston: McGraw-Hill Irwin; 2006.

17. Newstrom J. Leveraging management development through the management of transfer. J Manag Dev 1986;5(5):33–45.

18. Goldstein I, Ford J. Training in organizations. Belmont (CA): Wadsworth; 2002.

19. Baldwin T, Ford J. Transfer of training. Person Psychol 1988;41:63–105.

20. Clayton K, Blumberg F, Auld D. The relationship between motivation, learning strategies and choice of environment whether traditional or including an online component. Br J Educ Technol 2010;41(3):349–64.

21. Arthur W, Bennett W, Edens P, et al. Effectiveness of training in organizations: a meta-analysis of design and evaluation features. J Appl Psychol 2003;88(2): 234–45.

22. Blume B, Ford J, Baldwin T, et al. Transfer of training: a meta-analytic review. J Manag 2010;36(4):1065–91.

23. Cook D, Brydges R, Hamstra S, et al. Comparative effectiveness of technology-enhanced simulation versus other instructional methods: a systematic review and meta-analysis. Simul Healthc 2012;7:308–20.

24. Frengley R, Weller J, Torrie J, et al. The effect of a simulation-based training intervention on the performance of critical care unit teams. Crit Care Med 2011; 39(12):2605–11.

25. Buckley T, Gordon C. The effectiveness of high fidelity simulation on medical-surgical registured nurses' ability to recognise and respond to clinical emergencies. Nurse Educ Today 2011;31(7):716–21.

26. Goldsworthy S, Graham L. Simulation simplified: a handbook for nurse educators. Philadelphia: Lippincott; 2013.

27. Foronda C, Gattamorta K, Snowden K, et al. Use of virtual clinical simulation to improve communication skills of baccalaureate nursing students: a pilot study. Nurse Educ Today 2014;34:e53–7.

28. Cant R, Cooper S. Simulation-based learning in nurse education: systematic review. J Adv Nurs 2010;66(1):3–15.

29. International Nursing Association for Clinical Simulation and Learning (INACSL) (2013). Standards of Best Practice. Available at: http://www.nursingsimulation.org/issue/S1876–1399(13)X0013-1. Accessed June 1, 2016.

30. Ford D, Seybert A, Smithburger P, et al. The impact of simulation based learning on medication error rates in critically ill patients. Intensive Care Med 2010;36: 1526–31.

31. White A, Brannan J, Long J, et al. Comparison of instructional methods: cognitive skills and confidence level. Clin Simul Nurs 2013;9(10):e417–23.

32. Meyer M, Connors H, Hou Q, et al. The effect of simulation on clinical performance: a junior nursing student clinical comparison study. Simul Healthc 2011; 6(5):269–77.

33. Sears K, Goldsworthy S, Goodman W. The relationship between simulation and medication safety. J Nurs Educ 2010;49(1):52–5.

34. Facteau J, Dobbins G, Russell J, et al. The influence of general perceptions of training environment on motivation and perceived training transfer. J Manag 1995;21(1):1–25.

35. Goldsworthy S. The mechanisms by which professional development may contribute to Critical Care Nurses' intent to stay. Vancouver (Canada): University of British Columbia; 2015.

36. Schwarzer R, Jerusalem M. Generalized self-efficacy scale. In: Weinman J, Wright S, Johnston M, editors. Measures in health psychology: a user's portfolio.

Causal and control beliefs. Windsor (United Kingdom): NFER-NELSON; 1995. p. 35–7.

37. Goldsworthy S. High fidelity simulation in critical care: a Canadian perspective. Collegian 2012;19(3):139–43.

38. Goldsworthy S, Graham L. Compact clinical guide to mechanical ventilation: foundations of practice for critical care nurses. New York: Springer Publishing; 2014.

Early Mobilization of Mechanically Ventilated Patient

Pam Hruska, RN, MSc

KEYWORDS

- Early mobilization • Mechanical ventilation • Mobility • Critically ill
- Active mobilization • Passive mobilization • Progressive mobilization

KEY POINTS

- Critically ill patients requiring mechanical ventilation are least likely to be mobilized.
- Use of bed rest and oversedation in mechanically ventilated patients has likely been shaped from historical practices.
- Early mobilization of mechanically ventilated patients is safe and can lead to decreased time on the ventilator, reduced length of stay and improved functional mobility.
- Early mobilization of the mechanically ventilated patient should progress from passive to active interventions given evidence suggests both forms activity provide patient benefit.

INTRODUCTION

Mechanical ventilation has evolved dramatically since its advent in the early 1800s.[1] With each iteration of technology developed, patient-ventilator interactions have played a role in shaping the ability to mobilize patients receiving this type of therapy. Negative pressure ventilators, such as the iron lung used throughout the polio epidemic, encased a patient's entire body except for the head in a tubelike chamber. These types of ventilators allowed limited access to patients for provision of care and ingrained the use of prolonged bed rest.[1] Positive pressure ventilation, provided by way of an advanced artificial airway, has taken over since the 1940s and development of this more invasive form of mechanical ventilation initially required use of deep sedation to allow patients to tolerate therapy.[2]

At present, ICU ventilator development is in its fourth generation, and allows for the provision of a wide variety of ventilatory modes.[1] This has been important not only for improvement in the type of supports available for management of respiratory failure in the critically ill but also for providing the opportunity to nurse mechanically ventilated

The author has nothing to disclose.
Department of Critical Care Medicine, Alberta Health Services, 3134 Hospital Drive, Northwest Calgary, Alberta T2N 2T9, Canada
E-mail address: Pam.Hruska@ahs.ca

Crit Care Nurs Clin N Am 28 (2016) 413–424
http://dx.doi.org/10.1016/j.cnc.2016.07.002
0899-5885/16/Crown Copyright © 2016 Published by Elsevier Inc. All rights reserved.

patients differently from what was possible during the times of the iron lung or with strictly mandatory control modes of ventilation. Lessons learned throughout the evolution of mechanical ventilation have allowed us to reach a point in time where patient-ventilator interactions have improved so much that patients can tolerate this therapy without requiring deep sedation for many ventilatory modes via technology that has dramatically less physical restriction. These points are important to highlight, because one of the top-emerging concerns reported in current literature related to patient-ventilator interactions is how immobility and muscle loss in critically ill patients lead to long-term physical weakness and neuromuscular abnormalities, present in up to 95% of surviving patients at 5-year follow-up.[3–7]

Immobilization and mechanical ventilation linkages might best be exemplified by findings that those with endotracheal tubes (ETTs) are least likely to be mobilized or at risk for having limited mobilization until this interventional support is removed.[8–10] With mean estimates of 39.5% of patients requiring mechanical ventilation during any given hour in US critical care units,[11] emphasis on mobility in the intubated patient population is required. These estimated usages of ventilatory support are even low in some instances, as it has been demonstrated there is variable use of ventilators throughout North America, with rates even 20% to 40% higher in some Canadian ICUs.[12] The need for attention to this topic is reinforced by work that suggests it is likely that 1 in 16 go on to require prolonged mechanical ventilation due to complications of acquired weakness, leading to increased duration of patient stay.[6,13] Given the likelihood for immobility and prolonged complications from weakness is increased in mechanically ventilated patients, the purpose of this article is to provide a basic overview of the literature related to early mobilization in this at-risk patient population.

INACTIVITY AND TYPES OF WEAKNESS

Increased focus on long-term outcomes of critically ill patients has identified that physical inactivity and muscle weakness are common in those who have been in critical care and required mechanical ventilation.[3,4,14] Inactivity leading to weakness has been described in a few different ways in relation to both the diaphragm and skeletal muscles. The types of weakness described in literature are summarized in **Table 1** and are a result of different underlying mechanisms.

EARLY MOBILIZATION ACTIVITIES

The risk of developing critical illness neuromyopathies is as high as 50% in patients who have had sepsis, multiorgan failure, or prolonged mechanical ventilation.[17] Early mobility interventions aim to offset weakness by assisting patients in maintaining or restoring as much mobility and functional independence as possible. Activities used to accomplish these goals are typically determined by a patient's ability to participate and can include a wide range of options from simple passive repositioning to out-of-bed, active mobilization. Although not exhaustive in nature, **Box 1** provides a summary of activities used in early mobilization of critically ill patients. These activities are categorized as passive or active in nature. Passive mobilization activities are defined as movements performed without volitional control[18] and do not require active participation from a patient because they are performed by a provider or a device.[19] Active mobilization, on the other hand, requires patient participation and ranges from assisted support during mobilization to independent activity.[20]

Nydahl and colleagues[8] identified devices used to assist patients with early active mobilization to include special chairs, sliding boards, special beds, walkers, lifting devices, tilt tables, portable ventilators, and standing frames. Findings in relation to use

Table 1
Types of weakness

Type of Weakness	Definition
Deconditioning	Multiple changes in organ systems that are caused by inactivity, thought to occur within 4 h of bed rest[15]
Atrophy	Loss in net protein content and fat-free mass due to an imbalance between protein synthesis and protein degradation, leading to smaller and weaker muscles in both fast and slow muscle fibers[4]
Mechanical unloading	Decreased exposure to sustained mechanical loads on muscles leading to catabolism and depressed contractile function linked to the degradation of actin thin filaments; lessened force of the muscle in combination with atrophy leads to additive weakness[4]
Critical illness neuromyopathy	A syndrome that occurs in patients who have severe illness leading to disorder of the peripheral nerves, muscles and/or neuromuscular junction that develops during ICU stay[6]
Ventilator-induced diaphragmatic dysfunction	Damage to the lungs related to atrophy and contractile dysfunction of the diaphragm as a result of prolonged mechanical ventilation[5,16]

Data from Refs.[4–6,15,16]

Box 1
Early mobilization activities

Passive mobilization activities

- Supported range of motion[18]
- Stretching[21]
- Turns and repositioning in bed[20]
- Tilt table therapy[22]
- Specialty beds[22]
- Passive cycle ergometer[23]
- Neuromuscular electrical stimulation[24,25]

Active mobilization activities

- Participating with turns in bed[20]
- In-bed exercises, such as weights or cycling[20]
- Inspiratory muscle training/breathing exercises[24]
- Sitting and/or standing balance exercises at the side of the bed[20,24]
- Transferring to a chair[20]
- Marching at the bedside[20]
- Assisted ambulation[20]
- Independent ambulation[20]

Data from Refs.[18,20–25]

of these devices suggest patients were significantly more likely to be mobilized out of bed if a lift, standing frame and/or portable ventilator was present; however, in units with available specialty beds, patients were significantly less likely to be mobilized out of bed.[8] These findings imply that devices can be a double-edged sword for active mobilization. On the one hand, they help patients participate in activities that they otherwise could not achieve independently, whereas on the other hand, the devices may be items of convenience that may hinder full-mobility progression if overly depended on or incorrectly used.

SAFETY CONSIDERATIONS AND READINESS

Mobilizing critically ill patients requires assessment of the patient's physiologic reserve to determine how well activity might be tolerated. This is broadly done through a head-to-toe, systems-based approach and extensive lists of recommendations for safety criteria have been outlined in consensus documents informed by work previously done to investigate if early activity is safe for critically ill patients who require mechanical ventilation.[26–28] In addition to physical assessment, it is own important to gather information on how patients tolerate nursing interactions, patients' awareness of their emotional state and understanding of what patients' baseline level of activity was prior to hospitalization for decision making.[26] Delineating safety factors that are intrinsic to patients (their physiologic status) as well as factors extrinsic to patients (physical attachments, lines, tubes, environment, and staffing) is another structured way to approach assessing feasibility for mobilization.[26]

Inclusion criteria in some of the research investigating early mobilization established a priori that any patient unable to respond to verbal commands would not participate in interventions.[28] Exclusion of comatose patients may arguably omit a large percentage of the critically ill patient population and one way to include them is to consider assessment findings in context of whether mobilization is performed with passive or active activities.[27] Hodgson and colleagues[27] established an approach for safe mobilization by generating consensus recommendations in the form of a table with 4 main categories that providers should evaluate to determine readiness. These categories include respiratory considerations, cardiovascular considerations, neurologic considerations, and other considerations (ie, lines and tubes).[27] For each category of consideration, items listed within the table, such as the presence of an ETT or a respiratory rate of greater than 30, had an associated color-coded symbol using a traffic-light system for in-bed and out-of-bed exercises. With green implying little risk, yellow suggesting significant potential for risk, and red requiring communication with senior ICU staff prior to any mobilization, this system for assessment helps identify the potential for an adverse event.[27]

One item that lacks consensus is if patient dependence on inotropic or vasoactive medications for cardiovascular support is a contraindication for mobilization.[26–28] There is agreement that the use of inotropes and vasoactive medications should not be an absolute contraindication for early mobilization, but explicit dosages or changes in doses to be concerned about have not been defined. Instead, recommendations encourage conversations about appropriateness for mobilization in this patient group on a case-by-case basis.[26,27]

TIMING, DOSING, AND FREQUENCY

The timing, dosing and frequency of early mobilization activities are variable and have been identified as topics that require further investigation.[22,29] As previously discussed, some researchers only permitted early mobilization in patients who could follow commands,[28] whereas others established that passive mobilization, possible with stretching or electrical stimulating devices, helps prevent muscle atrophy.[21] Passive mobilization activities have potential for other benefits as well, such as maintenance of range of motion, prevention of contractures, maintenance of soft tissue length, and possible increased muscle stregnth.[18,19,23,25] In light of this, the appeal to redefine the description of mobility in critical care to be inclusive of both passive and active activities, which progress mobility along a continuum as patients tolerate,[30] should be supported.

MEASURING IMPACTS OF EARLY MOBILIZATION

Data from literature report on the impacts of early mobilization in a variety of ways and the more commonly used measures are summarized in **Table 2**. These measurement examples are organized into categories of patient outcomes, functional status, ratings on scales or tools, and health-related quality-of-life measures. Findings related to these measurements mostly afford insight into gross patient outcomes after they have left critical care and may not be sensitive enough to inform decision making while patients are still within the unit.

BENEFITS AND OUTCOMES OF EARLY MOBILIZATION

The previously discussed outcome measures have been helpful for demonstrating benefits of early mobilization. These benefits include decreased length of ICU and hospital stay as well as improvements in muscle strength and functional status.[31,37,38] From a functional standpoint, one interventional study found that 69% of patients treated with early mobilization were able to walk greater than 100 feet on ICU discharge.[28] Other studies have noted decreased duration of delirium days, decreased days of mechanical ventilation, and improved patient functional status.[20,31] Additionally, discharge rates to home (as opposed to care facilities) were improved with early mobilization.[20,38] Other novel findings associated with early mobilization interventions have described an increased need in the amount of opioids patients required, attributed to increased pain experienced with activity.[39] One metric explored, which may not be a sensitive indicator for identifying benefits of mobility interventions in research, was mortality outcomes. Data related to mortality at time of hospital discharge did not reflect any differences in on analysis of five different research studies.[20]

THE BARRIER OF SEDATION

Despite highlighted benefits of early mobilization, many barriers for being able to provide activity have been identified. One of the top-cited barriers to mobilizing critically ill patients is related to use of sedation.[10,22,40–42] Often used to maintain patients in a calm state,[22] sedation acts as a form of pharmacologic restraint that perpetuates prolonged bed rest and is reportedly used to prevent patient self-harm (ie, self-extubation).[40] With an increasing amount of evidence pointing out the harms of oversedation, such as ventilator-associated pneumonia[43] and how it contributes to long-term dysfunctions associated with immobility, attention directed at reducing use of these medications has been achieved with protocols that interrupt sedation daily.[44]

PERSPECTIVES RELATED TO USE OF SEDATION

Nurses described caring for nonsedated, mechanically ventilated patients as "demanding but rewarding," allowing for increased interaction between the nurse and patient that promoted person-centered care.[45] From a patient perspective, being mechanically ventilated with lightened or no sedation caused feelings of vulnerability, anxiousness, fear, and loneliness.[46] It also caused altered body image or distorted

Table 2
Measuring impacts of early mobilization in critically ill patients

Measurement	Description
Patient outcome	
Ventilator-free days	Number of ventilator-free days during the first 28 d of hospital stay[31]
Duration of ventilation	Average amount of time spent on a ventilator[22]
Length of stay	Defined as either the length of stay within ICU or in hospital, reported in days[20]
Mortality	Defined as either the mortality rates on hospital discharge, or at 1 y time[20]
Functional status	
Mean ambulation distance at ICU discharge	The distance the patient is able to walk assisted or unassisted, as measured in feet[28]
6-min walk test	The distance a patient can walk in 6 min on a flat surface[32,33]
Muscle strength	Assessed by measuring respiratory muscle force, upper and lower limbs muscle force, or hand-grip force[20]
Scales and tools	
Chelsea critical care physical assessment tool	A tool developed to assesses components of physical morbidity, including respiratory function, cough strength, moving within the bed, supine to sitting on the edge of the bed, dynamic sitting, standing balance, sit to stand, transferring from bed to chair, stepping, and grip strength[34]
Perme ICU Mobility Score	Used within a cardiovascular ICU, this tool scores 15 items grouped into 7 categories of mental status, potential mobility barriers, functional strength, bed mobility, transfers, gait, and endurance[35]
Barthel Index	A tool used to assess patients after ICU discharge that measures 10 different activities of daily living[32]
FIM	An 18-item tool proposed as an outcome measure for pulmonary rehabilitation. Of the 18 items, 13 assess motor ability and 5 assess cognitive ability.[36]
Physical function ICU test	Once a patient is able to sit out of bed, use of this tool captures the patient's ability for sit to stand, marching on the spot, shoulder flexion, and muscle strength.[32]
Health-related quality of life	
Return to work	Considered a proxy measure for functional status that lacks a consistent format[33]
Medical outcomes study 36-item short form	Captures 8 dimensions of health: physical functioning, role physical, bodily pain, general health, vitality, social functioning, and role emotion.[33]
EuroQol-5D	Assesses 5 domains of health: mobility, self-care, usual activities, pain or discomfort, anxiety, and depression[32]

Data from Refs.[20,22,31–36]

body awareness, attributed to having limited possibilities to act as a result of being restrained by the technology attached.[47] This led to feeling a lack of trust in one's body, being out of touch with reality and time, changed appearance, and a lack of control.[47] With this in mind, nursing availability for providing explanations and for developing emotionally supportive relationships was important from a patient point of view.[46] The amount of emotional support required in caring for these patients was achievable with 1:1 nurse-patient ratios,[45] and staffing assignments should consider how to factor in these patient needs. Patients have also expressed the importance of including relatives in their care to help them through the experience of being mechanically ventilated without sedation.[46] This sentiment is a shared one, because relatives thought that their deep relationship with critically ill patients could be of benefit for assisting the health care team in determining the need for sedation or pain control, for providing insight into interpreting patient responses, and for helping to be a positive impact by being a familiar voice.[48]

OTHER BARRIERS

In addition to sedation as a barrier, other barriers to early mobilization in mechanically ventilated patients identified include the presence of an ETT[10,49] neurologic impairment, hemodynamic and respiratory instability.[50] Mechanical ventilation via an ETT may even be a more pertinent issue within North America, because duration of intubation with this type of airway (as opposed to a tracheostomy) has been noted to be in place for almost twice as long as compared to patients cared for in Australia or Scotland.[10] Less common considerations include patient obesity and time restraints caused by increased expectations for the amount of required patient care and documentation.[22] When exploring barriers from a multidisciplinary perspective, it was mutually agreed on among physicians, physiotherapists, and nurses that the presence of an ETT, staffing concerns, and increased workload had an impact on patient activity. Suggested ways for overcoming these barriers included use of mobility teams, multidisciplinary team planning, senior level administrative support, and increased staff training about how to mobilize intubated patients.[49]

PERCEIVED RESPONSIBILITY

The perceived responsibility of who should initiate mobilization of critically ill patients makes a difference on if or when activity occurs. This phenomenon was uncovered in a grounded dimensional analysis by Doherty-King and Bowers,[51] during which they identified that nurses held divided opinions about if they were responsible for initiating mobilization or if this was best suited for another discipline, such as medicine or physiotherapy. Nurses who thought that initiating mobilization was within their responsibility were motivated to help patients regain independence and make a positive impact on the psychological well-being of the patients. In general, these nurses overcame potential barriers by being collaborative with physiotherapy, assessing appropriateness of orders, diminishing risk as best possible, and working within the confines of resources available.[51]

Nurses who thought it was the responsibility of a physician or physiotherapist to initiate mobilization preferred to defer decision making because they were concerned about potential for injury to the patient and waited for physiotherapy clearance, physician orders, a decrease in perceived risks, and resources to improve.[51] Furthermore, in nurses who thought it was a physician's responsibility to initiate mobilization, orders were often adhered to in a rigid manner, such that if an order indicated that a patient should be up in a chair three times per day, nurses would stick to this explicitly even if they thought the patient was able to achieve a higher level of activity.[51] This is important because if the trigger for mobilization hinges on an order, the way the order is written may need to encourage practice that communicates the need for mobilization to be progressive in nature so activity is not unnecessarily restricted.

ADMINISTRATIVE SUPPORT FOR EARLY MOBILIZATION

Some researchers have discussed perceptions about early mobilization in critically ill patients from an administrative point of view.[22] Morris[22] suggested there exists an administrative reluctance to invest in human labor for the purpose of early mobilization of critically ill patients; however, these comments may be speculative in nature and at present there is no evident literature that can be found directly asking administrators about their perspective. There is also the possibility administrators think there are enough human resources available to achieve mobility goals with the right adoption and change management strategies. Future research exploring this leadership perspective would be beneficial.

INTEGRATING MOBILITY INTO CARE

Integrating mobilization into the workflow processes for critical care within existing human resources available has been exemplified by work done by Mah and colleagues.[52] In an attempt to develop a feasible mobility program within critical care, this research considered all the steps that would have to happen to make mobilization possible. This approach outlined inclusion criteria for mobilization, required points of communication between health care professionals, expectations for rounding practices, expectations for mandatory functional evaluations within 48 hours of admission, and a guiding document for progressing patients through a stepwise activity protocol.[52] This detailed coordination of care led to significantly improved functional independence measure (FIM) scores in patients.[52] Other investigators have additionally credited implementation success to educational workshops and team collaboration.[53] Team composition in some implementations have suggested that in addition to existing registered nursing and respiratory therapy staff, a full-time physiotherapist is required to support early mobility.[54] These implementations did not seem to lead to negative impacts on unit culture as evidenced by high self-rated scores from staff related to climate of safety and teamwork.[55]

HOW TO MOBILIZE MECHANICALLY VENTILATED PATIENTS

Although the message about the need for early mobilization in mechanically ventilated patients is repeated frequently in literature, there seems to be a lack of resources outlining steps on how to mobilize mechanically ventilated patients. It is not unrealistic to assume it is intimidating to mobilize a critically ill patient; if unit culture of practice does not currently foster comfort with this skill, literature available to describe the precise steps for coordinating this activity is scarce.

ADVERSE EVENTS

Researchers who have conducted interventional mobilization research within critical care report few to no adverse events as a result of their protocols. Although it is prudent to be concerned about the potential for these risks, falls, dislodgement of catheters or tubes, and accidental removal of the ETT were not reported in a resource-efficient, mobilization program.[52] Systematic reviews tracking safety and feasibility provide further details about types of adverse events that have occurred, including situational hypertension and hypotension, oxygen desaturations, accidental extubation, arrhythmias, removal of feeding tubes or radial arterial lines, patient ventilator-asynchrony, and minor falls.[38] The percentages of adverse events reported ranged from 0% to 3.76%, demonstrating that mobilization with critical care patients carries a small amount of risk. When adverse events related to hemodynamic changes occurred, the situation resolved with rest and required minimal interventions from the medical team.[20]

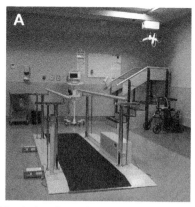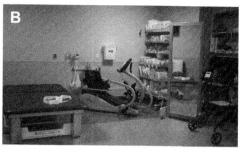

Fig. 1. (*A, B*) South Health Campus ICU gym, Calgary, Alberta, Canada.

PERIPHERAL PRACTICES

There are some key peripheral practices related to the topic of early mobilization that deserve attention and should be considered in tandem with efforts to improve mobilization within critical care units. These practices include consideration of the following:

- Fall-prevention practices
- Delirium assessment and management
- Sedation guidelines
- Nutrition
- Sleep hygiene

FUTURE STRATEGIES

Acknowledgment about the importance of early mobilization has led to evidenced-based design in newly built critical care units. This is highlighted by two ICUs in Calgary, Alberta, Canada, which have rehabilitation gyms within their units. **Figs. 1** and **2**

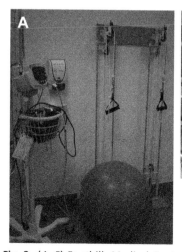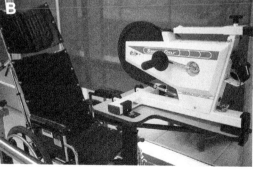

Fig. 2. (*A, B*) Foothills Medical Centre ICU gym, Calgary, Alberta, Canada.

capture examples of these designated spaces that provide nearby access to rehabilitation equipment.

SUMMARY

This article highlights the importance of early mobilization in mechanically ventilated patients and suggests this patient group is at risk for being least likely to be mobilized. Use of bed rest and overuse of sedation in this patient population are likely a result of historical practices related to patient-ventilator interactions; however, this literature review demonstrates mobility in this patient population is possible and safe. Assessing mobility readiness in context of progressing patients from passive to active activities can lead to long-term benefits and has been achievable with resource-efficient implementations and teamwork.

REFERENCES

1. Kacmarek RM. The mechanical ventilator: past, present, and future. Respir Care 2011;56(8):1170–80.
2. Marini J. Mechanical ventilation- past lessons and the near future. Crit Care 2013; 17(Suppl 1):10.
3. Truong AD, Fan E, Brower RG, et al. Bench-to-bedside review: mobilizing patients in the intensive care unit–from pathophysiology to clinical trials. Crit Care 2009;13(4):216.
4. Chambers MA, Moylan JS, Reid MB. Physical inactivity and muscle weakness in the critically ill. Crit Care Med 2009;37(10 Suppl):S337–46.
5. Powers SK, Kavazis AN, Levine S. Prolonged mechanical ventilation alters diaphragmatic structure and function. Crit Care Med 2009;37(10 Suppl):S347–53.
6. De Jonghe B, Lacherade JC, Durand MC, et al. Critical illness neuromuscular syndromes. Crit Care Clin 2007;23(1):55–69.
7. Skinner EH, Berney S, Warrillow S, et al. Rehabilitation and exercise prescription in Australian intensive care units. Physiotherapy 2008;94(3):220–9.
8. Nydahl P, Ruhl AP, Bartoszek G, et al. Early mobilization of mechanically ventilated patients: a 1-day point-prevalence study in Germany. Crit Care Med 2014;42(5):1178–86.
9. Berney S. Intensive care unit mobility practices in Australia and New Zealand: a point prevalance study. Crit Care Resusc 2013;15(4):260–5.
10. Harrold ME, Salisbury LG, Webb SA, et al. Early mobilisation in intensive care units in Australia and Scotland: a prospective, observational cohort study examining mobilisation practises and barriers. Crit Care 2015;19:336.
11. Wunsch H, Wagner J, Herlim M, et al. ICU occupancy and mechanical ventilator use in the United States. Crit Care Med 2013;41(12):2712–9.
12. Rapoport J, Teres D, Barnett R, et al. A comparison of intensive care unit utilization in Alberta and western Massachusetts. Crit Care Med 1995;23(8):1336–46.
13. Lorne N, Walsh T. Prolonged mechanical ventilation in critically ill patients- epidemiology, outcomes and modelling the potential cost consequences of establishing a regional weaning unit. Crit Care 2011;15(R102):1–10.
14. De Jonghe B, Sharshar T, Lefaucheur JP, et al. Paresis acquired in the intensive care unit a prospective multicenter study. JAMA 2002;288:2859–67.
15. Winkelman C. Inactivity and inflammation in the critically ill patient. Crit Care Clin 2007;23(1):21–34.
16. Petrof BJ, Jaber S, Matecki S. Ventilator-induced diaphragmatic dysfunction. Curr Opin Crit Care 2010;16(1):19–25.

17. Stevens RD, Dowdy DW, Michaels RK, et al. Neuromuscular dysfunction acquired in critical illness: a systematic review. Intensive Care Med 2007;33(11):1876–91.
18. Stockley RC, Hughes J, Morrison J, et al. An investigation of the use of passive movements in intensive care by UK physiotherapists. Physiotherapy 2010; 96(3):228–33.
19. Stockley RC, Morrison J, Rooney J, et al. Move it or lose it? A survey of the aims of treatment when using passive movements in intensive care. Intensive Crit Care Nurs 2012;28(2):82–7.
20. Li Z, Peng X, Zhu B, et al. Active mobilization for mechanically ventilated patients: a systematic review. Arch Phys Med Rehabil 2013;94(3):551–61.
21. Griffiths R. Effect of passive stretching on the wasting of muscle in the critically ill. Nutrition 1997;13:4.
22. Morris PE. Moving our critically ill patients: mobility barriers and benefits. Crit Care Clin 2007;23(1):1–20.
23. Dos Santos LJ, de Aguiar Lemos F, Bianchi T, et al. Early rehabilitation using a passive cycle ergometer on muscle morphology in mechanically ventilated critically ill patients in the Intensive Care Unit (MoVe-ICU study): study protocol for a randomized controlled trial. Trials 2015;16(1):383.
24. Choi J, Frederick T, Hoffman L. Mobility interventions to improve outcomes in patients undergoing prolonged mechanical ventilation- a review of the literature. Biol Res Nurs 2008;10(1):12.
25. Kho ME, Truong AD, Zanni JM, et al. Neuromuscular electrical stimulation in mechanically ventilated patients: a randomized, sham-controlled pilot trial with blinded outcome assessment. J Crit Care 2015;30(1):32–9.
26. Stiller K. Safety issues that should be considered when mobilizing critically ill patients. Crit Care Clin 2007;23(1):35–53.
27. Hodgson CL, Stiller K, Needham DM, et al. Expert consensus and recommendations on safety criteria for active mobilization of mechanically ventilated critically ill adults. Crit Care 2014;18(6):658.
28. Bailey P, Thomsen GE, Spuhler VJ, et al. Early activity is feasible and safe in respiratory failure patients. Crit Care Med 2007;35(1):139–45.
29. Castro-Avila AC, Seron P, Fan E, et al. Effect of early rehabilitation during intensive care unit stay on functional status: systematic review and meta-analysis. PLoS One 2015;10(7):e0130722.
30. Makic MB. Rethinking mobility and intensive care patients. J Perianesth Nurs 2015;30(2):151–2.
31. Schweickert W, Pohlman M, Pohlman A, et al. Early physical and occupational therapy in mechanically ventilated, critically ill patients- a randomised controlled trial. Lancet 2009;373:8.
32. Elliott D, Denehy L, Berney S, et al. Assessing physical function and activity for survivors of a critical illness: a review of instruments. Aust Crit Care 2011;24(3):155–66.
33. Hayes J, Black N, Jenkinson C, et al. Outcome measures for adult critical care- a systematic review. Health Technol Assess 2000;4(24):1–111.
34. Corner EJ, Wood H, Englebretsen C, et al. The Chelsea critical care physical assessment tool (CPAx): validation of an innovative new tool to measure physical morbidity in the general adult critical care population; an observational proof-of-concept pilot study. Physiotherapy 2013;99(1):33–41.
35. Nawa RK, Lettvin C, Winkelman C, et al. Initial interrater reliability for a novel measure of patient mobility in a cardiovascular intensive care unit. J Crit Care 2014; 29(3)(475):e471–5.

36. Montagnani G, Vagheggini G, Panait Vlad E, et al. Use of the Functional Independence Measure in people for whom weaning from mechanical ventilation is difficult. Phys Ther 2011;91(7):1109–15.
37. Schweickert WD, Kress JP. Implementing early mobilization interventions in mechanically ventilated patients in the ICU. Chest 2011;140(6):1612–7.
38. Cameron S, Ball I, Cepinskas G, et al. Early mobilization in the critical care unit: a review of adult and pediatric literature. J Crit Care 2015;30(4):664–72.
39. Witcher R, Stoerger L, Dzierba AL, et al. Effect of early mobilization on sedation practices in the neurosciences intensive care unit: a preimplementation and post-implementation evaluation. J Crit Care 2015;30(2):344–7.
40. Hofso K, Coyer FM. Part 1. Chemical and physical restraints in the management of mechanically ventilated patients in the ICU: contributing factors. Intensive Crit Care Nurs 2007;23(5):249–55.
41. Kress JP. Sedation and mobility: changing the paradigm. Crit Care Clin 2013; 29(1):67–75.
42. Gosselink R, Needham D, Hermans G. ICU-based rehabilitation and its appropriate metrics. Curr Opin Crit Care 2012;18(5):533–9.
43. Clemmer TP. Why the reluctance to meaningfully mobilize ventilated patients? "The answer my friend is blowin' in the wind". Crit Care Med 2014;42(5):1308–9.
44. Hofso K, Coyer FM. Part 2. Chemical and physical restraints in the management of mechanically ventilated patients in the ICU: a patient perspective. Intensive Crit Care Nurs 2007;23(6):316–22.
45. Laerkner E, Egerod I, Hansen HP. Nurses' experiences of caring for critically ill, non-sedated, mechanically ventilated patients in the Intensive Care Unit: a qualitative study. Intensive Crit Care Nurs 2015;31(4):196–204.
46. Baumgarten M, Poulsen I. Patients' experiences of being mechanically ventilated in an ICU: a qualitative metasynthesis. Scand J Caring Sci 2015;29(2):205–14.
47. Johansson L, Fjellman-Wiklund A. Ventilated patients' experiences of body awareness at an intensive care unit. Adv Physiother 2015;7(4):154–61.
48. Dreyer A, Nortvedt P. Sedation of ventilated patients in intensive care units: relatives' experiences. J Adv Nurs 2008;61(5):549–56.
49. Barber EA, Everard T, Holland AE, et al. Barriers and facilitators to early mobilisation in Intensive Care: a qualitative study. Aust Crit Care 2015;28(4):177–82.
50. Garzon-Serrano J, Ryan C, Waak K, et al. Early mobilization in critically ill patients: patients' mobilization level depends on health care provider's profession. PM R 2011;3(4):307–13.
51. Doherty-King B, Bowers BJ. Attributing the responsibility for ambulating patients: a qualitative study. Int J Nurs Stud 2013;50(9):1240–6.
52. Mah JW, Staff I, Fichandler D, et al. Resource-efficient mobilization programs in the intensive care unit: who stands to win? Am J Surg 2013;206(4):488–93.
53. Bassett RD, Vollman KM, Brandwene L, et al. Integrating a multidisciplinary mobility programme into intensive care practice (IMMPTP): a multicentre collaborative. Intensive Crit Care Nurs 2012;28(2):88–97.
54. Clark DE, Lowman JD, Griffin RL, et al. Effectiveness of an early mobilization protocol in a trauma and burns intensive care unit: a retrospective cohort study. Phys Ther 2013;93(2):186–96.
55. Hopkins RO, Spuhler VJ, Thomsen GE. Transforming ICU culture to facilitate early mobility. Crit Care Clin 2007;23(1):81–96.

Optimizing Oxygenation in the Mechanically Ventilated Patient

Nursing Practice Implications

Glenn Barton, MSN (Ed), RN[a],*,
Brandi Vanderspank-Wright, PhD, RN, CNCC(C)[b],
Jacqueline Shea, MScN, RN[c]

KEYWORDS

- Critical care nursing • Mechanical ventilation • Oxygenation • Patient safety
- Hypoxia

KEY POINTS

- Critical care nurses must possess advanced knowledge, skill, and judgment when implementing and evaluating oxygenation improvement strategies with mechanically ventilated patients.
- Effectively communicating findings of the nursing assessment and patient response to oxygenation interventions are integral to informing ongoing patient treatment decisions.
- Nurses in the intensive care unit are well-positioned to anticipate, monitor, and prevent complications related to invasive and potentially risky oxygen improvement therapies.

INTRODUCTION

Most critical care interventions target the optimization of end organ oxygenation to some degree. Hypoxia is frequent grounds for admission to the intensive care unit (ICU), carrying with it high patient acuity and demands for complex interventions such as positive pressure mechanical ventilation.[1] When hypoxic patients are admitted to the ICU, critical care nurses maintain a continuous therapeutic presence with them and mounting literature suggests that these nurses are playing an increasingly active role specific to oxygenation and mechanical ventilation.[2,3] Recent studies

No conflicts to declare.
[a] Department of Practice, Performance and Innovation, Health Systems Innovation and External Relations, Royal College of Physicians and Surgeons of Canada, 774 Echo Drive, Ottawa, Ontario K1S 5N8, Canada; [b] Faculty of Health Sciences, School of Nursing, University of Ottawa, 3245B Roger Guindon Hall, 451 Smyth Road, Ottawa, Ontario K1H 8M5, Canada; [c] Surgery, The Ottawa Hospital, General Campus, 450 Smyth Road, Ottawa, Ontario K1H 8M5, Canada
* Corresponding author.
E-mail address: gbarton@royalcollege.ca

highlight the need to more critically evaluate the overall risk–benefit associated with oxygen improvement strategies, and that potentially the hypoxia problem is being overtreated.[4,5] In their role, ICU nurses not only require knowledge to appropriately implement oxygen treatment measures, they also demand competent skill and judgment to anticipate, monitor, and intervene when complications arise.

Improving oxygenation in the ventilated patient is widely studied; however, this literature rarely targets a nursing practice audience.[6] Furthermore, terms used to quantify and communicate clinical oxygenation parameters can be confusing, complicated, and controversial.[7] Given requirements for clinical information that is clear and consistent, it is essential that ICU nurses possess the communicative capacity required to best relay their holistic knowledge related to patient oxygenation status.

This article provides insight into several best practice nursing considerations for optimizing oxygenation in ventilated patients. We first situate the topic by providing an overview of relevant principles pertaining to gas exchange and measurement. We then clarify some frequently used clinical terms. Common rescue therapies used to optimize oxygenation in ventilated patients are described, including patient positioning, ventilatory strategies, and pharmacologic measures. Informed by our recent review of the literature, discussion in this article emphasizes findings of practical relevance for ICU nurses, specifically direct nursing care implications for patients receiving these therapies, particularly where they intersect with issues related to patient safety.

UNDERSTANDING AND COMMUNICATING OXYGENATION PRINCIPLES

Nearly 3% of hospital stays in the United States involve mechanical ventilation[8] and the primary reason for both adult and pediatric ICU admission is complex respiratory support.[9] Knowledge of pulmonary gas exchange and indices used to measure it are fundamental to the critical care nursing role. Oxygenation is facilitated through inspiration or positive pressure ventilation when intubated as air is dispersed through pressure and laminar flow from central airways out to the alveoli.[10] Here, in the lung's functional units gas is dissolved into blood as available oxygen molecules diffuse rapidly through a thin complex interface of alveolar epithelium and surrounding pulmonary capillaries. Red blood cells flowing tightly through these capillaries also bind to oxygen as the prime delivery mechanism for transport throughout the body.[10] Preventing hypoxemia (impaired pulmonary gas exchange) relates directly to ensuring sufficient alveolar O_2 supply is available for diffusion and also that sufficient capillary blood volume and flow at this exchange interface is maintained.

Basic oxygenation measures such as PaO_2, SaO_2, and SpO_2 are often discussed but can be used erroneously in clinical dialogue. It is therefore important to define and highlight distinctions between these common terms often used to quantify oxygenation status. These measures often serve as endpoints determining whether interventions to improve oxygenation are successful; however, these indices merely reflect effectiveness of pulmonary gas exchange and oxygen available for delivery rather than providing direct measure of appropriate oxygenation at the tissue level.[11]

PaO_2 refers to a global measurement specific to the partial pressure of oxygen dissolved in blood plasma. The normal range of PaO_2 is 80 to 100 mm Hg.[12] Conversely, SaO_2 is a measurement expressed as percentage of available oxygen bound to hemoglobin with a normal range of 95% or greater to 100%.[12] Nearly 98% of oxygen available for tissue delivery is found bound to hemoglobin with the remaining 2% dissolved in blood plasma.[10] Ellstrom (2006) notes that "[a]rterial oxygenation is considered compromised when [hemoglobin] saturation is less than 88% (PaO_2 [less than]

60 mm Hg)."[13] Both PaO_2 and SaO_2 are acquired through arterial blood gas sampling. SpO_2, while also providing a measurement of oxygen saturation, is readily available through noninvasive pulse oximetry. The normal reference range for SpO_2 is 95% or greater; however, targets for SpO_2 vary depending on a patient's underlying pathophysiology and preexisting comorbidities. Hypoxia (impaired tissue oxygenation) occurs as a result of hypoxemia caused by deficiencies of the respiratory system and/or mechanisms of oxygen delivery (ie, cardiac output, hemoglobin level).[14] Critical care nurses are well-positioned as direct care providers to use their competency with these principles and measurement indices to comprehensively inform decision making of the health care team.

Ventilation–Perfusion Mismatch

As mentioned, disproportionate relationships between oxygen supply (ventilation) and blood supply (perfusion) around alveoli can cause hypoxemia (PaO_2 <60 mm Hg) and without intervention, hypoxia.[14] In a normal respiratory unit (ie, 1 functional alveoli and corresponding capillary bed with good flow), oxygen and carbon dioxide diffuse across the alveolar membrane with ease. However, units can become impaired resulting in altered ventilation–perfusion (V/Q) mismatch (**Fig. 1**). In a dead space unit, ventilation remains normal (functional alveoli) but perfusion is impaired. Causes of this "high" V/Q mismatch may include pulmonary embolism or cardiogenic shock.[13,15] In this instance, clinical interventions to maintain adequate oxygenation are aimed at treating underlying issues with perfusion (see Promoting Hemodynamic Stability). In the inverse situation, where the problem lies with ventilation and perfusion is normal (ie, shunt unit),

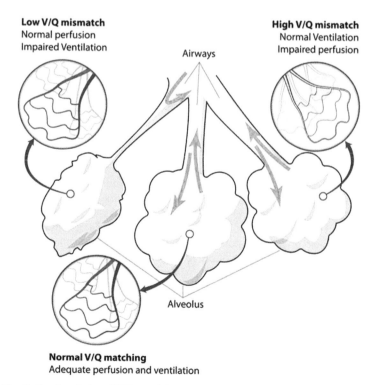

Low V/Q mismatch
Normal perfusion
Impaired Ventilation

Airways

High V/Q mismatch
Normal Ventilation
Impaired perfusion

Alveolus

Normal V/Q matching
Adequate perfusion and ventilation

Fig. 1. Ventilation/perfusion (V/Q) matching.

blood passing through the pulmonary capillary cannot pick up oxygen from a poorly functioning (or nonfunctioning) respiratory unit. Causes of this "low" V/Q mismatch include atelectasis, pneumonia, and pulmonary edema. In this instance, interventions can be aimed at improving oxygenation through management of ventilator parameters (ie, increasing positive end-expiratory pressure [PEEP] or using alveolar recruitment measures; see Positive End-expiratory Pressure and Recruitment Maneuvers), determining optimal patient positioning (ie, lateral semirecumbent positions or prone positioning; see Patient Positioning), as well as adequate suctioning and airway management. In silent units, both ventilation and perfusion are affected. Interventions in this instance are aimed at optimizing both ventilation and perfusion. In addition, intrapulmonary shunt is the body's own adaptive mechanism attempting to minimize V/Q mismatch. Intrapulmonary shunt refers to localized capillary vasoconstriction resulting in bypass of blood to better ventilated areas.[16] Occurring in response to low alveolar PaO_2, this compensatory response elicits constriction of pulmonary arterial vessels, minimizing wasted perfusion, and promoting gas exchange at functional respiratory units. Improving V/Q mismatches when they exist is a common goal of all modalities used to improve oxygenation in the mechanically ventilated patient.

THE NURSING ROLE IN OPTIMIZING OXYGENATION IN THE MECHANICALLY VENTILATED PATIENT

The nursing role and process with respect to optimizing oxygenation encompasses advanced assessments, planning, implementation and evaluation of interventions. Although, manipulating ventilatory settings such as PEEP or oxygen concentration can be carried out to meet patient needs, these are not necessarily first-line interventions nurses might consider to address low oxygen levels. Recent systematic reviews[17,18] provide this nursing perspective, describing critical thinking processes and strategies adopted when a ventilated patient presents with new onset respiratory or cardiac instability.[17]

Core Components of Respiratory Assessment

Nursing respiratory assessment of the intubated patient while holistic in nature has specific components related directly to oxygenation and mitigating threats to patient safety. In the mechanically ventilated patient, verification of ventilatory parameters including settings and alarms should be completed, including SpO_2 and respiratory rate alarms normally set on the cardiac monitor. In performing a respiratory assessment, the critical care nurse should also consider respiratory rate, work of breathing, and lung sounds in addition to objective measures of oxygenation including PaO_2 values, SaO_2, SpO_2, as well as the patient's tidal and minute volumes. Presence of dyspnea, asynchronous chest and abdominal movements, use of accessory muscles, and agitation should all be indicators of potential oxygenation problems and also the need to reassess appropriateness of present ventilator settings.[19]

Airway Patency and Placement

Nursing practice decisions related to oxygenation in mechanically ventilated patients, also focus on assessing and verifying airway patency and endotracheal tube (ETT) placement.[17] This assessment includes ensuring that the airway is secured properly and verifying the airway insertion length.[17] Strategies used to verify ETT placement include use of end-tidal carbon dioxide monitoring with capnometry and capnography.[20] Both capnometry and capnography have been found to be reliable methods of verification in addition to radiological examination via chest radiograph.[21]

Verification of airway patency can be accomplished by assessing for obstruction in the ETT and the presence of lung secretions. Patients who are ventilated mechanically are at risk of developing secretions because mechanical ventilation bypasses humidification and filtration of the upper airways occurring with normal respiration and, furthermore, intubated patients are unable to clear secretions independently.[22] Therefore, the presence of secretions is assessed through performance of endotracheal suctioning. Verification of tube patency and placement ensures that the system of delivering oxygen is properly in situ and that patient harm from unplanned extubation and upper airway obstruction are minimized.

Endotracheal suctioning enables the nurse to assess color, consistency, and amount of secretions, which in turn supports oxygenation through the removal of obstructive residue,[23] potentially causing low V/Q mismatch. It is important to assess how the patient responds to this procedure (ie, does the patient's SpO_2 decrease or does suctioning negatively impact other vital signs?). Critical care nurses need to be aware of the negative effects of endotracheal suctioning. Suctioning should not be performed routinely (eg, q4h) to limit the possibility of adverse events.[17] Although evidence suggests suctioning should be done on an as-needed basis, the intervention can be valuable for reducing consolidation–atelectasis risk, thus promoting oxygenation in the ventilated patient.[24] Caution should also be exercised owing to the risks associated with endotracheal suctioning such as bleeding, infection, atelectasis, hypoxemia, cardiovascular instability, increased intracranial pressure, and trauma to the tracheal mucosa.[24] When deciding to suction for oxygenation benefits, nurses need to consider individual patient illness and condition while critically evaluating these potential risks in the ventilated patient.

Nursing practice recommendations related to suctioning include using a catheter less than one-half the diameter of the ETT lumen with the lowest continuous negative pressure possible for less than 15 seconds.[24] During suctioning, catheters should not be advanced past the carina, aseptic technique should be followed, and saline lavage avoided.[24] Particularly fragile patients should be hyperoxygenated before and after the suction procedure and provided hyperinflation combined with hyperoxygenation on a nonroutine basis.[24] Assessment of a patient's ventilator settings, changing FiO_2 requirements, PaO_2, heart rate, mean arterial pressure, and period of time for SpO_2 recovery should all be considered by the assigned health professional.[17] These assessment findings can provide insight into the patient's present respiratory condition, potentially signaling oxygenation deterioration or improvement.

Pharmacologic Assessment and Intervention

Assessing sedation–analgesic requirements needed to decrease work of breathing or facilitate comfort with intubation are also nursing concerns related to optimizing oxygenation. These traumatic factors often occurring in mechanically ventilated patients result in unnecessary stress response and catecholamine surge, inducing states of decreased supply and increased oxygen demand.[25] A patient's level of consciousness and comfort level should be evaluated using evidence-based tools such as the validated Richmond Agitation and Sedation Scale and Critical Care Pain Observation Tool.[26,27] Using sedation–analgesia can also assist with complications related to ventilator dyssynchrony or a patient fighting the vent; facilitating maximum therapeutic oxygenation benefits provided by the ventilator.

Neuromuscular blocking agents are another important pharmacologic intervention used by nurses to manage hypoxia in the ventilated patient. These drugs facilitate gas exchange by reducing extrapulmonary resistance and ventilator dyssynchrony associated with severe lung injury. Paralysis of skeletal muscle such as the diaphragm allows for metabolic rest and reduced oxygen consumption, and allowing for complete mechanized control over breathing mechanics. Evidence suggests that patients receiving neuromuscular blocking agents for adult respiratory distress syndrome (ARDS) require less PEEP to maintain oxygenation targets,[28] and have reduced mortality to hospital discharge compared with control groups.[28,29] Regardless of the potential oxygenation benefits that pharmacologic measures may provide, nurses assessing and administering these drug therapies should follow established best practice guidelines, and reducing the well-documented patient risks such as ICU delirium, prolonged mechanical ventilation, and ICU-induced myopathy.[30]

Patient Positioning

Patient positioning for therapeutic benefit has long been identified as a primary nursing responsibility. Patient position examples used in critical care settings include supine, semirecumbent, side lying, and prone. The most common position supported by evidence is the semirecumbent position with the head of the bed elevated between 30° and 45° to reduce risk of developing ventilator-acquired pneumonia.[31] Positions found to be useful in improving oxygenation among intubated patients include right or left side lying (lateral decubitus) and prone position.[32,33] Misasi and Keyes[34] (1996) stressed the importance of nurses taking into account relevant lung pathology when positioning the ICU patient population. For example, positioning a mechanically ventilated patient in a side lying position with affected lung up can improve oxygenation for patients with unilateral lung disease.[34] It is also suggested that altering the critically ill patient's position can shorten ICU duration of stay and improve the patient's outlook for recovery.[34]

Prone Positioning

Proning is a carefully coordinated positioning intervention that involves placing the mechanically ventilated patient in a face down, backside up posture[32,33] resulting in oxygenation improvements at least 70% of the time.[1,35] The maneuver has been studied most extensively in patients with ARDS and in this population is thought to improve oxygenation–ventilation–perfusion relationships by recruiting increased alveoli in outer dorsal regions of the lung, allowing for more even distribution of tidal volume delivered and improving secretion drainage and ventilation to dependent lung areas.[1,35]

Although a recent systematic review suggests proning provides no mortality benefit in ARDS patients,[1] there are subpopulations for whom the position confers great benefit. These include those patients most severely hypoxemic, those who are proned early (within 48 hours of ARDS diagnosis), and those who remain prone for at least 16 hours per day.[1] Knowledge of these benefits is useful for critical care nurses with respect to early advocacy and preparation for prone positioning in their patients.

The majority of serious adverse events reported in the proning literature relate to the actual maneuver itself and it is suggested that a majority of these can be prevented and treated with excellent nursing care.[35] Airway obstruction from ETT kinks and ETT displacement, including accidental extubation while turning, can be minimized through standardized protocols followed by experienced and well-coordinated nursing teams. To mitigate lost airway risks, 1 person should be designated to monitor and maintain the security of the ETT. This same person should call out steps in the turning sequence similar to a leader monitoring body alignment when coordinating a log roll in a patient with C-spine injury. Final positioning of the patient's head allowing for easy view and access to the oropharynx could also be helpful in mitigating airway displacement (**Fig. 2**). Frequent oral suctioning and meticulous mouth care can minimize retained oral secretions and therefore reduce saliva leakage that degrade the

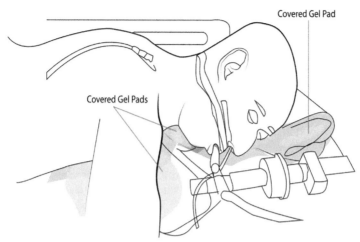

Fig. 2. Facial pressure relief and airway visualization with prone position. Position the head appropriately on gel pad–covered linens to visualize the airway, and prevent pressure ulceration and ocular nerve compression associated with facial edema.

viscous integrity of ETT securement devices. Hemodynamic instability and cardiac arrhythmia are also described as potential complications and attention should be brought to anticipating any prompt titration, or need to initiate vasoactive drugs should hemodynamic instability persist. Electrocardiographic electrodes can be placed posteriorly on the patient's back and similarly anterior/posterior placement of defibrillator pads considered should cardiac arrest occur.

Retinal nerve compression, profound facial swelling, and decubitus ulcers are well-documented complications associated with prone positioning.[1,35] Facial ulceration may be especially prevalent on the cheeks, forehead, and orbital regions. As with all skin care strategies, attentive monitoring, frequent repositioning, and minimizing not easily visible moisture collections with use of dry linens or absorbable pads can be beneficial.[36] Strategic placement of gel pads or padded rolls at identified pressure points are also helpful (see **Fig. 2**). Meticulous nursing care is the preventative measure for a majority of complications that can ensue after a decision to prone a patient.

Promoting Hemodynamic Stability

Nurses play a pivotal role in managing patient respiratory status, and this includes anticipating collateral hemodynamic effects associated with interventions used to facilitate oxygenation. For example, seemingly inert tasks such as lowering the head of bed may affect cardiac function and ultimately blood flow and/or perfusion. Any intervention that predominantly increases intrathoracic pressure can result in reduced cardiac preload because venous return is affected negatively. Increased intrathoracic pressure can occur during suctioning, patient positioning, and particularly with high PEEP settings. Preexisting cardiovascular compromise might also dictate how much impact mechanical ventilation has on the patient's venous return and cardiac status.[37] Consequently, nurses need to assess, anticipate, and implement interventions to manage these effects. Their assessment should include observing for complications associated with poor cardiac output. This includes pre–post comparative evaluation of the patient's heart rate, cardiac rhythm, blood pressure, central venous pressure, peripheral perfusion, urine output, chest radiograph, and serum electrolytes.[17,38] These monitoring and evaluation practices can reduce the risk of cardiac output impairment for these patients.[37] To this end, it is important that perfusion and not just ventilation be prioritized, because interventions and practices promoting adequate blood flow to tissues correspondingly promote oxygenation.

Positive End-Expiratory Pressure and Recruitment Maneuvers

Nursing knowledge of ventilatory strategies used to improve oxygenation in critical illness is also important. It is beyond the scope of this paper to discuss ventilation modes specific to oxygenation improvement however, we felt it necessary to discuss 2 common rescue interventions specific to the ventilator.

PEEP is a constant pressure maintained in the ventilator circuit that promotes oxygenation by facilitating diffusion and recruiting collapsed alveoli, thus increasing surface area available for gas exchange.[39] Therefore, making PEEP adjustments regardless of ventilator mode has a direct impact on a patient's oxygenation status. Although higher PEEP levels have been associated with improved mortality benefits in patients with life-threatening hypoxemia, debate over what constitutes an optimal PEEP target still exists.[39]

Recruitment maneuvers improve oxygenation by providing brief but sustained inspiratory flow cycles to a maximum plateau pressure, also inflating collapsed alveoli.[40] Optimal circumstances, target plateau pressure, and time period for which to apply recruitment maneuvers is again controversial.[41] Although it is suggested that these maneuvers provide temporary increases to oxygenation by PaO_2 measurement, the improvements are not sustained, and furthermore do not provide a statistically significant benefit to patient-centered outcomes such as mortality and number of ventilation days.[41] Given this lack of evidence, recruitment maneuvers should most likely not be part of routine care and are probably best reserved as rescue therapy for severe refractory hypoxemia or after accidental disconnection from ventilator.

Despite the recognized oxygenation benefits of recruitment maneuvers and higher PEEP level, there are also risks for nurses to consider. Both of these ventilator driven therapies increase peak airway pressures, increasing risk of barotrauma (pressure related damage) and volutrauma (volume related damage) in the lungs.[40] In addition, these applications increase intrathoracic pressure and, as mentioned, can have detrimental hemodynamic effects (ie, hypotension, arrhythmia) by impairing venous return and increasing right ventricular afterload.[40,42] Close monitoring of any such hemodynamic and respiratory effects when ventilator adjustments are made is required by nurses to mitigate increased threats of patient harm.

SUMMARY

ICU nurses play a major role in caring for the ventilated patient with compromised oxygenation status. Given nursing's responsibility for implementing oxygenation interventions, evaluating these, and communicating patient response to the team, it is essential that they possess a skilled understanding and communicative capacity to discuss complex respiratory issues and oxygenation monitoring parameters. Nursing aptitude with this knowledge is integral to informing good clinical decisions made by the health care team.

Although commonplace in critical care settings, treatment modalities used to optimize oxygenation are not without risk. Given their continuous presence with the patient, ICU nurses are well-positioned to monitor for complications, and mitigate iatrogenic threats to patient safety. Instituting treatment strategies to blindly improve oxygenation parameters in the event of respiratory decline risks narrow-minded practice. Much like attending to the intricate balance of oxygen supply and demand, interprofessional health care leaders need always consider holistic risk–benefit analysis for any ICU intervention.

REFERENCES

1. Bloomfield R, Noble D, Sudlow A. Prone position for acute respiratory failure in adults. Cochrane Database Syst Rev 2015;(11):CD008095.
2. Blackwood B, Junk C, Lyons J, et al. Role responsibilities in mechanical ventilation and weaning in pediatric intensive care units: a national survey. Am J Crit Care 2013;22(3):189–97.
3. Rose L, Ramagnano S. Emergency nurse responsibilities for mechanical ventilation: a national survey. J Emerg Nurs 2013;39(3):226–32.
4. Helmerhorst H, Roos-Blom M, van Westerloo D, et al. Association between arterial hyperoxia and outcome in subsets of critical illness. Crit Care Med 2015; 43(7):1508–19.
5. Panwar R, Hardie M, Bellomo R, et al. Conservative versus liberal oxygenation targets for mechanically ventilated patients: a pilot multicenter randomized controlled trial. Am J Respir Crit Care Med 2016;193(1):43–51.
6. Graham L, Goldsworthy S. Compact clinical guide to mechanical ventilation: foundations of practice for critical care nurses. New York: Springer Publishing Company; 2014.
7. Lemaire F. Thematic session on acute respiratory failure. Gas exchange in mechanically ventilated patients: definition of ARDS: is oxygenation a good index? Program and abstracts of the 15th Annual Congress of the European Society of Intensive Care Medicine. Barcelona, Spain, September 29–October 2, 2002.
8. Wunsch H, Linde-Zwirble W, Angus D, et al. The epidemiology of mechanical ventilation in the United States. Crit Care Med 2010;38(10):1947–53.
9. Critical care statistics. Critical care patients. Society of Critical Care Medicine. Available at: http://www.sccm.org/Communications/Pages/CriticalCareStats. aspx. Accessed May 25, 2016.
10. Pittman RN. Regulation of tissue oxygenation. San Rafael (CA): Morgan & Claypool Life Sciences; 2011.
11. Benedik PS, Hamlin SK. Monitoring tissue blood flow and oxygenation: a brief review of emerging techniques. Crit Care Nurs Clin North Am 2014;26(3):345–56.
12. Barry M, Goldsworthy S, Goodridge D. Medical-surgical nursing in Canada: assessment and management of clinical problems. 3rd edition. Toronto: Elsevier; 2014.
13. Ellstrom K. The pulmonary system. In: Alspach JG, editor. AACN core curriculum for critical care nurses. 6th edition. St Louis (MO): Saunders Elsevier; 2006. p. 45–183.
14. Bein T, Grasso S, Moerer O, et al. The standard of care of patients with ARDS: ventilatory settings and rescue therapies for refractory hypoxemia. Intensive Care Med 2016;42(5):699–711.
15. St. John RE, Seckel MA. Airway and ventilatory management. In: Burns SM, editor. AACN essentials of critical care nursing. 3rd edition. New York: McGraw-Hill; 2014. p. 119–57.
16. Swenson ER. Hypoxic pulmonary vasoconstriction. High Alt Med Biol 2013;14(2): 101–10.

17. Couchman B, Wetzig S, Coyer F, et al. Nursing care of the mechanically ventilated patient: what does the evidence say? Intensive Crit Care Nurs 2007;23(1):4–14. Available at: http://bit.ly/GrammarlyB.

18. Coyer F, Wheeler M, Wetzig S, et al. Nursing care of the mechanically ventilated patient: what does the evidence say? Intensive Crit Care Nurs 2007;23(2):71–80.

19. Hillman K, Bishop G. Clinical intensive care and acute medicine. Cambridge (United Kingdom): Cambridge University Press; 2004.

20. DeBoer S, Seaver M, Arndt K. Verification of endotracheal tube placement. J Emerg Nurs 2003;29(5):444–50.

21. Grmec Š. Comparison of three different methods to confirm tracheal tube placement in emergency intubation. Intensive Care Med 2002;28(6):701–4.

22. St. John R, Malen J. Contemporary issues in adult tracheostomy management. Crit Care Nurs Clin North Am 2004;16(3):413–30.

23. Winters A, Munro N. Assessment of the mechanically ventilated patient. AACN Clin Issues 2004;15(4):525–33.

24. Pederson C, Rosendahl-Nielsen M, Hjermind J, et al. Endotracheal suctioning of the adult intubated patient-what is the evidence? Intensive Crit Care Nurs 2009; 25(1):21–30.

25. Papazian L, Forel J, Gacouin A, et al. Neuromuscular blockers in early acute respiratory distress syndrome. N Engl J Med 2010;363(12):1107–16.

26. Wesley E, Truman B, Ayum S, et al. Monitoring sedation status over time in ICU patients. JAMA 2003;289(22):2983–91.

27. Gelinas C, Johnston C. Pain assessment in the critically ill ventilated adult: validation of the Critical-Care Pain Observation Tool and physiologic indicators. Clin J Pain 2007;23(6):407–505.

28. Gainnier M, Roch A, Forel J, et al. Effect of neuromuscular blocking agents on gas exchange in patients presenting with acute respiratory distress syndrome. Crit Care Med 2004;32(1):113–9.

29. Alhazzani W, Alshahrani M, Jaeschke R, et al. Neuromuscular blocking agents in acute respiratory distress syndrome: a systematic review and meta-analysis of randomized controlled trials. Crit Care 2013;17(2):R43.

30. MacIntyre NR. Supporting oxygenation in acute respiratory failure. Respir Care 2013;58(1):142–50.

31. Bonten M. Prevention of hospital-acquired pneumonia: European perspective. Infect Dis Clin North Am 2003;17(4):773–84.

32. Drahnak D, Custer N. Prone positioning of patients with acute respiratory distress syndrome. Crit Care Nurse 2015;35(6):29–37.

33. Gibson K, Dufault M, Bergeron K. Prone positioning in acute respiratory distress syndrome. Nurs Stand 2015;29(50):34–9.

34. Misasi R, Keyes J. Matching and mismatching ventilation and perfusion in the lung. Crit Care Nurse 1996;16(3):23.

35. Gattinoni L, Taccone P, Carlesso E, et al. Prone position in acute respiratory distress syndrome. Rationale, indications, and limits. Am J Respir Crit Care Med 2013;188(11):1286–93.

36. The National Pressure Ulcer Advisory Panel - NPUAP. Prevention and treatment of pressure ulcers: clinical practice guideline. 2014. Available at: http://www.npuap. org/resources/educational-and-clinical-resources/prevention-and-treatment-of-pressure-ulcers-clinical-practice-guideline/. Accessed May 15, 2016.

37. Pinsky M. Cardiovascular issues in respiratory care. Chest 2005;128(5):592S–7S.

38. McGrath A, Cox C. Cardiac and circulatory assessment in intensive care units. Intensive Crit Care Nurs 1998;14(6):283–7.

39. Gattinoni L, Carlesso E, Cressoni M. Selecting the 'right' positive end-expiratory pressure level. Curr Opin Crit Care 2015;21(1):50–7.

40. Slutsky AS, Ranieri VM. Ventilator-induced lung injury. N Engl J Med 2013; 369(22):2126–36.

41. Hodgson C, Keating JL, Holland AE, et al. Recruitment manoeuvres for adults with acute lung injury receiving mechanical ventilation. Cochrane Database Syst Rev 2009;(2):CD006667.

42. Fan E, Wilcox ME, Brower RG, et al. Recruitment maneuvers for acute lung injury: a systematic review. Am J Respir Crit Care Med 2008;178:1156–63.

Best Practices for Managing Pain, Sedation, and Delirium in the Mechanically Ventilated Patient

Kitty M. Garrett, RN, MSN, CCRN, CCNS

KEYWORDS

- Sedation • Agitation • Pain • Delirium • Mechanical ventilation
- SCCM clinical practice guidelines • PAD Bundle • ABCDEF Bundle

KEY POINTS

- Prolonged sedation increases the risk of delirium. Delirium can lead to long-term neurocognitive deficits. Nurses play a crucial role in early recognition and possible prevention.
- Preventive measures proven to be effective include maintaining light levels of sedation, minimizing the use of benzodiazepines, decreasing ventilator time, and promoting early progressive mobility.
- Every patient should be screened/assessed at least once a shift for pain, agitation, and delirium, using valid and reliable assessment tools.
- Implementation of the PAD or ABCDEF bundle is recommended for use in every critical care nursing unit.
- All necessary resources for bundle implementation are available for unrestricted use in patient care and provider education on the icudelirium.org Web site.

INTRODUCTION

Management of pain, agitation, and delirium in the mechanically ventilated patient remains one of the biggest challenges in critical care nursing today. Nursing care priorities include strategies to minimize the physical and psychological discomfort and unpleasant memory associated with endotracheal intubation and mechanical ventilation. For decades, it was considered best practice to administer high doses of sedation and/or neuromuscular paralysis to maximize patient comfort and ventilator tolerance. In the late 1990s, several studies demonstrated negative patient outcomes of deep sedation, such as prolonged mechanical ventilation and increased risk of

Disclosure Statement: The author has nothing to disclose.
Department of Physiological and Technological Nursing, College of Nursing, Augusta University, 987 St. Sebastian Way, Augusta, GA 30912, USA
E-mail address: kigarrett@augusta.edu

Crit Care Nurs Clin N Am 28 (2016) 437–450
http://dx.doi.org/10.1016/j.cnc.2016.07.004
0899-5885/16/© 2016 Elsevier Inc. All rights reserved.

ventilator-associated pneumonia (VAP).[1,2] This knowledge led to the development of nurse-driven sedation scales and recommendations for daily wake-ups to lighten sedation levels and allow accurate neurologic assessments.[3–5] Research interest in this topic has continued to grow, and a review of the literature reveals a plethora of recently published evidence-based recommendations for management of pain, agitation, and delirium in mechanically ventilated patients. There is now undisputed evidence to support lighter levels of sedation to not only prevent VAP, but also other serious consequences, such as delirium, hazards of immobility, and prolonged hospital stays.[6,7]

This article provides a historical perspective of the management of pain, agitation, and delirium, and disseminates information contained in the guidelines (Society for Critical Care Medicine Clinical Practice Guidelines for the management of pain, agitation and delirium in adult patients in the intensive care unit) to promote their implementation in day-to-day nursing care. It is not intended to be an all-inclusive review, but rather a summary of major recommendations relevant to nursing practice. The reader is referred to the original clinical practice guidelines for a more thorough understanding of the recommendations and their levels of evidence.[8] Although the guidelines are not specific to mechanically ventilated patients, they address issues relevant to this patient population.

SOCIETY FOR CRITICAL CARE MEDICINE GUIDELINES/PAIN, AGITATION, AND DELIRIUM BUNDLE

In January of 2013, the Society for Critical Care Medicine (SCCM) published clinical practice guidelines for the management of pain, agitation, and delirium in adult patients in the intensive care unit (ICU).[8] The guidelines were revised from a previously published version in 2002.[9] They differ from the previous guidelines in that all recommendations are evidence-based, rather than being based on expert opinion or consensus statements. They incorporate current research findings relative to improved methods of patient assessment and best practices regarding the pharmacologic and nonpharmacologic treatment of pain, agitation, and delirium. They are also intended to be less prescriptive in that, unless strongly supported by research, they recommend personalized approaches to choice of medications used.

Among 20 authors of the guidelines, five were critical care nurses who had an equal voice in contributing to the guideline content and revisions. The input of these nurses helped provide insight into the unique challenges of nursing care, enhancing the value of the guidelines in everyday critical care nursing practice. The new guidelines incorporate recommendations for more intense interprofessional collaboration and communication, impacting day-to-day nursing care of the mechanically ventilated patient more than ever before.[10]

To consolidate findings into a workable tool for implementation, the 2013 guidelines led to the creation of the PAD (pain, agitation, and delirium) Bundle. The PAD Bundle consists of 32 recommendations and 22 summary statements. The Bundle emphasizes an integrated approach to assessment, treatment, and prevention of significant pain, oversedation or undersedation, and delirium in critically ill patients. The guidelines recommend the use of specific nursing assessment tools, which have been proven to be the most valid and reliable measurement instruments for pain, agitation, and delirium. There are separate tools for assessment of each problem (pain, agitation, and delirium) to minimize ambiguity so that there is no temptation to oversedate patients to cover all three problems. Although pain, agitation, and delirium are addressed individually, it is recognized that they are not isolated problems but interrelated (**Table 1**).

PAIN: HISTORICAL PERSPECTIVE

Adult ICU patients routinely experience pain at rest and with routine ICU care, such as turning, endotracheal suctioning, procedures, or wound care.[11] Inadequate treatment of pain leads not only to unnecessary suffering, but complications, such as impaired mobility, prolonged ventilator time, psychological stress, and possible delirium.[12] Self-reporting is the gold standard for assessment of pain.[12,13] In critically ill patients who are able to communicate, the numeric rating scale has been shown to be the most valid and reliable for measuring intensity of pain.[13–15] This well-known and commonly used pain scale measures the intensity of pain from 0 to 10, with zero being no pain and 10 being the worst imaginable pain. However, this is a challenge in mechanically ventilated patients because of the presence of the endotracheal tube and the patient's sedation-induced altered level of consciousness.[16] Vital signs have not been found to correlate with either patient's self-report of pain or behavioral pain scores. But because they may change with pain, distress, or other factors, they are a cue to perform further pain assessment in patients.[17]

In a position statement published by the American Society for Pain Management, Herr and coworkers[17] addressed several populations of patients unable to self-report pain. Providing quality and compassionate care to patients who cannot self-report their pain is directed by the principle of justice, defined as the equal or comparative treatment of individuals. Respect for human dignity is the first principle of the American Nursing Association Code of Ethics, which directs nurses to advocate for humanity and give appropriate care.[17] The author reminds nurses that that all persons with pain deserve prompt recognition and treatment. Pain should be routinely assessed, reassessed, and documented to facilitate treatment and communication among health care clinicians.

A hierarchical approach to pain assessment is recommended by Pasero and McCaffery.[18] In patients who are unable to self-report, the nurse should search for potential causes of pain. These may include recent surgery, trauma, injury, infections, invasive lines/tubes, or painful procedures. The nurse should use a pain scale to observe patient behaviors. Next, the authors suggest using proxy reporting, which means that a family member or other person close to the patient can contribute to the assessment by knowing what is normal behavior for the patient. A trial of analgesia should then be attempted.[18]

The pain scales found to be the most reliable and valid in nonverbal patients are the Behavioral Pain Scale, created by Payen and coworkers in 2001[19] to identify unique behaviors in mechanically ventilated patients presented with noxious stimuli, and the Critical Care Pain Observation Tool.[20] The Critical Care Pain Observation Tool includes evaluation of four different behaviors (facial expressions, body movements, muscle tension, and compliance with the ventilator for mechanically ventilated patients or vocalization for nonintubated patients).

SEDATION/AGITATION: HISTORICAL PERSPECTIVE

It is recognized that most mechanically ventilated patients require some level of sedation, at least initially after intubation. Factors such as the presence of an endotracheal tube, the inability to speak, the dyssynchrony of controlled breaths, and the frequent need for physical restraints have been shown to contribute to patient discomfort in mechanically ventilated patients. For years, nurses kept patients "comfortable" by administering high doses of sedatives and neuromuscular blockers to enhance ventilator tolerance.[21] As long as the patient was hemodynamically stable, this was thought

Table 1
ICU PAD Bundle

	Pain	Agitation	Delirium

Assess	Assess pain ≥4 times/shift and prn
	Preferred pain assessment tools:
	  Patient able to self-report → NRS (0–10)
	  Unable to self-report → BPS (3–12) or
	    CPOT (0–8)
	Patient is in significant pain if NRS ≥4,
	  BPS >5, or CPOT ≥3
		Assess agitation. sedation ≥4 times/shift
		  and prn
		Preferred sedation assessment tools:
		  RASS (−5 to +4) or SAS (1–7)
		  NMB → suggest using brain function
		    monitoring[a]
		Depth of agitation, sedation defined as:
		  Agitated if RASS = +1 to +4, or SAS = 5–7
		  Awake and calm if RASS = 0, or SAS = 4
		  Lightly sedated if RASS = −1 to −2, or
		    SAS = 3
		  Deeply sedated if RASS = −3 to −5 or
		    SAS = 1–2
			Assess delirium every shift and prn
			Preferred delirium assessment tools:
			  CAM-ICU (+or -)
			  ICDSC (0–8)
			Delirium present if:
			  CAM-ICU is positive
			  ICDSC ≥4

Treat	Treat pain within 30′ then reassess:
	Nonpharmacologic treatment: relaxation
	  therapy[b]
	Pharmacologic treatment:
	  Nonneuropathic pain → IV
	    opioids ± nonopioid analgesics
	  Neuropathic pain → gabapentin or
	    carbamazepine, + IV opioids
	  S/p AAA repair, rib fractures → thoracic
	    epidural
		Targeted sedation or DSI (goal: patient
		  purposely follows commands without
		  agitation): RASS = −2 - 0, SAS = 3–4
		If under sedated (RASS >0, SAS >4) assess/
		  treat pain → treat w/sedatives prn
		  (nonbenzodiazepine[c] preferred, unless
		  ETOH or benzodiazepine withdrawal is
		  suspected)
		If over sedated (RASS <-2, SAS <3) hold
		  sedatives until at target, then restart at
		  50% of previous dose
			Treat pain as needed
			Reorient patients; familiarize surroundings;
			  use patient's eyeglasses, hearing aids if
			  needed
			Pharmacologic treatment of delirium:
			  Avoid benzodiazepines unless ETOH or
			    benzodiazepine withdrawal is suspected
			  Avoid rivastigmine
			  Avoid antipsychotics if increased risk of
			    torsades de pointes

| Prevent | Administer preprocedural analgesia and/or nonpharmacologic interventions (eg, relaxation therapy)
 Treat pain first, then sedate | Consider daily SBT, early mobility and exercise when patients are at goal sedation level, unless contraindicated
 EEG monitoring if:
 At risk for seizures
 Burst suppression therapy is indicated for increased ICP | Identify delirium risk factors: dementia, HTN, ETOH abuse, high severity of illness, coma, benzodiazepine administration
 Avoid benzodiazepine use in those at increased risk for delirium
 Mobilize and exercise patients early
 Promote sleep (control light, noise; cluster patient care activities; decrease nocturnal stimulation)
 Restart baseline psychiatric medications, if indicated |

[a] Auditory evoked potentials, Bispectral Index, Narcotrend Index, Patient State Index, or State Entropy.

[b] Especially for chest tube removal.

[c] Propofol for use in intubated/mechanically ventilated patients and dexmedetomidine for use in either intubated or nonintubated patients.

Abbreviations: AAA, abdominal aortic aneurysm; BPS, Behavioral Pain Scale; CAM-ICU, Confusion Assessment Method for the ICU; CPOT, Critical-Care Pain Observation Tool; DSI, daily sedation interruption (also referred to as Spontaneous Awakening Trial); EEG, electroencephalography; ETOH, ethanol; ICDSC, ICU Delirium Screening Checklist; ICP, intracranial pressure; IV, intravenous; NMB, neuromuscular blockade; NRS, Numeric Rating Scale; RASS, Richmond Agitation and Sedation Scale; SAS, Sedation-Agitation Scale; SBT, Spontaneous Breathing Trial.

Reproduced with permission from Barr J, Fraser GL, Puntillo K, et al. Clinical practice guidelines for the management of pain, agitation and delirium in adults patients in the intensive care unit. Crit Care Med 2013;41(1):294. Copyright © 2013 the Society of Critical Care Medicine and Lippincott Williams & Wilkins.

to be a safe practice. Benzodiazepines, such as lorazepam or midazolam, were frequently used.

Since that time, several studies have confirmed that prolonged sedation, ventilator time, and extended length of ICU stay lead to poor patient outcomes. Earlier studies focused on decreasing ventilator days to decrease the risk of VAP. In 1996, Ely and colleagues[22] published a landmark study related to spontaneous breathing trials (SBTs). They found that daily screening of the respiratory function of adults receiving mechanical ventilation followed by trials of spontaneous breathing in appropriate patients decreased ventilator time and possible ventilator complications. In 2000, Kress and colleagues[3] conducted another landmark study that confirmed the benefits of sedation vacations. They found that daily interruption of sedative drug infusions in mechanically ventilated patients decreased the duration of mechanical ventilation and length of stay in ICU. This was called the "spontaneous awakening trial" (SAT). These studies led to changes in practice related to lighter sedation as part of the recommended VAP bundle to prevent VAP. Nurses were encouraged to use nurse-driven sedation scales, such as the Sedation Assessment Scale[4] or the Richmond Agitation Sedation Scale,[5] as assessment tools for sedation titration. The Sedation Assessment Scale and the Richmond Agitation Sedation Scale are the most valid and reliable scales for assessing quality and depth of sedation in critically ill patients.[4,5] The purpose of sedation scales is to sedate the patient just enough to tolerate the ventilator without becoming too unresponsive.

The SAT Protocol and VAP Bundle are evidence-based, time-honored, and have been endorsed by critical care professional organizations for years. A growing body of evidence demonstrates that sedation protocols that minimize depth of sedation along with weaning protocols and early mobility protocols improve clinical outcomes, including shorter duration of ventilation and ICU stays. However, there continued to be evidence that patients were still being oversedated.[21] Critical care nurses are often reluctant to participate in daily awakening trials. They fear that patients may become frightened on awakening and self-extubate, remove invasive lines, or become combative.[21]

Although use of a sedation scale minimizes subjectivity among nursing staff, there may be differences in what is considered light sedation. Also, such factors as hemodynamic instability, organ dysfunction, or drug interactions may influence nursing judgment. Studies have shown that if there is any ambiguity, nurses tend to lean toward maximizing patient comfort with oversedation.[21] The new guidelines are more specific in the goal of "allowing patient responsiveness and awareness demonstrated by the ability to purposefully respond to commands."[8] It is hoped that this alleviates any clinical misperceptions of what is considered light sedation.

In 2008 Girard and coworkers[23] from Vanderbilt University published a study describing findings from a multicenter trial linking the efficacy and safety of minimizing sedation and mechanical ventilation days. They linked SATs with SBTs and collectively called this the Awakening and Breathing Controlled (ABC) Trial, using a protocol called Wake Up and Breathe. The Wake Up and Breathe protocol included safety screens for the SAT and the SBT, followed by a trial to assess patient readiness to wean (**Fig. 1**).

Findings were that those with paired SATs/SBTs had fewer days on the ventilator, shorter ICU and hospital lengths of stay, shorter duration of delirium/coma, and decreased long-term neuropsychological complications. Other benefits included an ability to more accurately titrate sedation, decreased incidence of VAP, and decreased need for neurologic testing related to oversedation.[23]

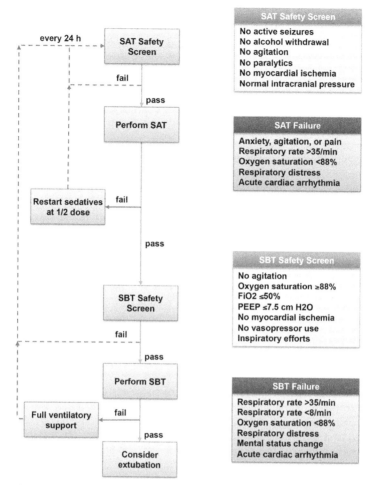

Fig. 1. Wake Up and Breathe protocol. SATs plus SBTs. FiO2, fraction of inspired oxygen; PEEP, positive end-expiratory pressure. (*Courtesy of* Vanderbilt University.)

This landmark study integrated the nurse's role in sedation management (sedation vacations) with the respiratory therapist's role in ventilator management (weaning), and led to many additional studies related to the prevention of oversedation and prolonged ventilation. Later studies revealed other benefits from lighter sedation, in addition to prevention of VAP.[24]

Regarding choice of sedative, the use of benzodiazepines is discouraged because of their long half-lives, which delay patient awakening. Dexmedetomidine and propofol are more appropriate agents for quicker awakening.[25] Benzodiazipines still remain important in the treatment of anxiety, seizures, and alcohol or benzodiazepine withdrawal.[8]

Early mobilization tends to have the most positive correlation thus far with a decreased incidence of delirium. Schweikert and coworkers in 2009 recognized that ICU patients with prolonged bedrest were prone to develop muscle weakness. They found that a program of whole-body mobility combined with lighter sedation led to more ventilator-free days, a decreased duration of delirium, and better neurologic functional outcomes.[26] Additional studies validated these findings, and progressive mobility is now recommended for all patients. Progressive mobility starts out with active range of motion, progresses to sitting up in bed, dangling, standing, transferring to a chair, and ambulating as tolerated.[27] More detailed information can be found in Pam Hruska's article, "Early Mobilization of Mechanically Ventilated Patient," in this issue.

DELIRIUM: HISTORICAL PERSPECTIVE

Delirium is defined as a "disturbance of consciousness with reduced ability to focus, sustain or shift attention, which develops over a short period of time and involves a change in cognition." It is designated as either hyperactive, defined as "agitated, disoriented and delusional with possible vivid hallucinations," or hypoactive, defined as "subdued, quietly confused, disoriented and apathetic."[28] The hyperactive form is less common (less than 2%) and less worrisome. The hypoactive form is seen in greater than 40% patients and is frequently missed. It has a far worse long-term prognosis because of decreased recognition, increased risk of reintubation, and mortality.[29] It leads to higher morbidity, increased ventilator days, longer hospital stays, and higher costs. Worst of all, it leads to long-term deterioration of cognitive and functional processes. A person who is delirious is unable to think clearly and cannot make sense of what is going on around them. Not only is this frustrating for patients and caregivers, but it delays patient participation in the recovery process. Poor functional recovery can persist for months after discharge; studies have been done up to 1 year after discharge.[29]

In the past, the occurrence of delirium in ICU patients was referred to as "ICU psychosis" and was attributed to prolonged ICU stays. Patients who were delusional or agitated would be treated with larger doses of sedatives and/or physical restraints, which led to more disorientation. There was also no ideal drug for this syndrome, although haloperidol was the drug prescribed most often. There was no clear-cut upper dosage limit of haloperidol; the more agitated the patient, the higher the dose. Nurses were encouraged to administer the drug until the patient became behaviorally managed, as long as hemodynamics and respiratory status were stable. Although haloperidol has been recommended as the preferred agent for the treatment of delirium, there is no published evidence that it prevents or reduces the duration of delirium in adult ICU patients.[8] The topic of delirium was not thought to be a serious concern and therefore, not well-studied. It was accepted that once the patient was transferred out of critical care and reoriented to a more normal environment, the syndrome would resolve.

In the last decade, there has been an increased awareness of the incidence of this ICU-induced psychosis. It has been found that delirium does not always resolve spontaneously and may indeed persist for months.[30–32] Studies have confirmed a high incidence of ICU patients who survive and recover from their physical conditions but spend months in rehabilitation because of a decline in cognitive function. This cognitive decline includes such symptoms as memory loss, decreased executive functioning, and weakness leading to falls. The risk of delirium in mechanically ventilated patients is high (60%–85%) and increases with each day of sedation and immobilization.[8,29] In addition to cognitive and memory problems, one-fourth of patients also report signs of posttraumatic stress disorders with terrifying flashbacks and hallucinations similar to those exposed to combat situations. Delusions can last long after discharge.

Delirium is underrecognized and underdiagnosed 80% of the time,[33] especially the hypoactive type. Symptoms of extreme sleepiness, inattention, and apathy are often missed with routine bedside assessment. Unfortunately, many patients with this syndrome have mistakenly been diagnosed as having dementia. The longer the duration of the delirium, the better predictor of cognitive impairment. So there is a need to recognize predisposing, precipitating factors. Because there are no obvious physical indicators, diagnosis relies on early astute assessment skills of the bedside caregiver. Although the underlying physiologic cause of delirium is still unknown, recent studies have led to an increase in knowledge of risk factors, prevention, and recognition. Risk factors include pre-existing dementia, history of hypertension, history of alcoholism, and a high severity of illness at admission. It is now known that delirium may be predictable and preventable through proactive interventions.[8,34]

Studies show that delirium is often triggered by large doses of antianxiety drugs and narcotics, especially in the elderly.[34] Other factors are hospital environments (busy, noisy, brightly lit) and hospital routines (sleep disruption caused by frequent vital signs, laboratory draws, laboratory studies, turning). In 2001, Ely and coworkers[35] developed an assessment tool for delirium called the Confusion Assessment Method for ICU patients (CAM-ICU), which was adopted from an earlier non-ICU version.[36] The CAM-ICU assesses the four main features of delirium to determine whether the patient is positive for delirium. The patient is positive for delirium if the onset is acute or fluctuating in course, the patient is inattentive, and either has altered level of consciousness or disorganized thinking. A CAM-ICU worksheet facilitates this assessment.[36]

Another assessment tool is the Intensive Care Delirium Screening Checklist (ICDSC).[37] The ICDSC is an eight-item checklist of delirium symptom evaluation over an 8- to 24-hour period. Symptoms include level of consciousness, inattention, disorientation, hallucination or delusion or psychosis, psychomotor agitation or retardation, inappropriate speech or mode, sleep/wake cycle disturbances, or symptom fluctuation.

The CAM-ICU and ICDSC delirium monitoring tools are the most valid and reliable scales to assess delirium in ICU patients.

THE ABCDEF BUNDLE

In his follow-up care of patients who survived ICU and mechanical ventilation, Dr. Wes Ely, from Vanderbilt University Medical Center, noted that frequently his patients, although fully recovering from their physical symptoms, showed signs of cognitive decline even months after their hospital discharge. He conducted several studies leading to many publications and a practice protocol for identification and treatment of delirium. Ely and his study group at Vanderbilt expanded the previously published ABC protocol to an ABCDE protocol. Slight changes were made to the ABC mnemonic, a "D" was added for "delirium", and an "E" was added for "early mobility." The new bundle was titled the Awakening and Breathing Coordination, Delirium Monitoring and Management and Early Mobility bundle. The ABCDE Bundle includes the same evidence-based recommendations for assessment, treatment, and prevention of pain, agitation, and delirium as the SCCM PAD Bundle. The goals of lighter sedation, attention to delirium, and early mobility are the same.[38] It is simply an alternately formatted tool intended to be helpful in operationalizing the PAD guidelines.

An "F" was later added to the bundle by investigators at Vanderbilt for "family engagement and empowerment" to help keep patients and families at the center of focused care. It was recognized that good communication with the patient's family is critical, and that empowering the family to be part of the team helps improve patient experiences. The meanings of the mnemonic A, B, and C changed slightly again, and

Box 1
Implications for nursing practice

1. Review of the SCCM PAD guidelines is recommended for every critical care nursing unit. The Vanderbilt Web site (icudelirium.org) offers unrestricted use of tools and education necessary to implement the PAD/ABCDEF Bundles.

2. Use screening assessments for pain, sedation, and delirium. Incorporate assessment tools into electronic documentation, order sets, and flowcharts.

3. Treat pain promptly and treat pain before sedating patient. Pain can promote delirium. If the patient remains agitated after treating, use bolus sedation dosing as needed initially. If frequent boluses are required (>3), use continuous intravenous sedation.[8]

4. Turn off sedation daily and restart only if needed at the lowest dose to maintain the chosen target level of consciousness. The goal is to lighten sedation to titrate to the patient's needs, not to simply withdraw the sedation. Always do what is best for the patient, not easiest for the nurse.

5. Avoid the use of benzodiazepines if possible. Dexmedetomidine or propofol are preferred agents for sedation. If atypical antipsychotics are indicated, monitor electrocardiogram accordingly to assess for risk of torsades de pointes.

6. Orient patients daily and engage them in conversation as much as possible. Screen for delirium. It patient is delirious, first seek reversible causes using the THINK mnemonic and attempt nonpharmacologic management.

7. Use nonpharmacologic methods to maximize rest periods, soften the environment, and encourage natural sleep/wake cycles. Darken the patient's room. Provide soothing music or white noise. Minimize interruptions to provide at least 4 hours of sleep at night. Do not wake patient up every 2 hours to check vital signs, check blood sugar, or reposition. Ensure that machines are not malfunctioning and alarming, and respond promptly to nuisance alarms. Allow patient to use eyeglasses and hearing aids. Use therapeutic touch. Try to decrease use of restraints. Provide high-quality compassionate nursing care.[41]

8. Develop a protocol that incorporates early progressive mobility and exercise for all critically ill patients.

9. An interdisciplinary ICU team approach is crucial. Nurses need to collaborate with respiratory therapists regarding optimum sedation scale goals and times for daily sedative interruption and breathing trials. Physical and occupational therapists should also be included in the plan of care so that patients are awake enough to participate in early progressive mobility efforts. Ideally, the interdisciplinary team should have consensus on individual sedation goals and make daily rounds to reassess as needed.

10. Coordinated care is essential; much interdisciplinary training needs to be done. A physician or nursing champion with knowledge of the research is helpful. To cooperate fully, nurses need to understand rationales for changes in practice. Administration should be included in the education process because of the possible need for extra staffing to accomplish the necessary goals.[38]

11. Data need to be kept and outcomes reported on sedation levels, time from intubation to mobility, ventilation days, delirium duration, and discharge disposition.[38]

12. Engage the family in patient care. Communication with the family is critical at every step of a patient's clinical course. Empowering the family to be part of the team helps ensure the best care for the patient.

Data from Refs.[8,38,41]

the bundle is currently referred to as the ABCDEF Bundle. The most updated version of the ABCDEF Bundle, according to the Vanderbilt Web site,[39] is as follows:

A: Assess for and manage pain
B: Both SATs and SBTs performed
C: Choice of sedation and analgesia
D: Delirium monitoring and management
E: Early mobility
F: Family engagement

To help address early identification of possible causes of delirium, the acronym THINK was created:

T: Toxic situations (heart failure, shock, dehydration, organ failure, and drugs)
H: Hypoxemia
I: Infection or sepsis/immobilization
N: Nonpharmacologic interventions used (eyeglasses, hearing aids, reorientation, sleep protocols, noise control)
K: K+ or other electrolyte problems

Ely and his ICU Delirium and Cognitive Impairment Study Group at Vanderbilt University Medical Center have developed an educational Web site relative to the recognition, symptoms, monitoring, and management of pain, agitation, and delirium.[39] The Web site includes detailed definitions, explanations, and examples of all components of the ABCDEF bundle. As leaders in delirium research, Vanderbilt is committed to education and global implementation of the SCCM recommendations. The Web site includes valuable resources for medical professionals, including copies of research articles, a timeline of landmark events in the history of delirium research, and copies of all nursing assessment tools with videotaped case studies demonstrating their use. There is also a section with articles and case studies specific for patients and families.

Although the ABCDEF Bundle is complex, successful implementation benefits the sickest patients the most. It improves communication among ICU team members, standardizes care processes, and breaks the cycle of oversedation and prolonged mechanical ventilation that can subsequently lead to delirium and weakness. The bundle helps to keep patients and families at the center and focus of care. Outcomes of mechanically ventilated patients are improved if the interventions described in the ABCDEF approach are used together as a bundle.[40]

See **Box 1** provides information regarding the implications for nursing practice.

SUMMARY

The 2013 ICU PAD guidelines provide critical care providers with an evidence-based, integrated, and interdisciplinary approach to managing pain, agitation/sedation, and delirium. The guidelines focus on those areas in which evidence is available to support the measures, specifically minimizing the use of benzodiazepines, maintaining light levels of sedation, and early mobility. Although there is no Food and Drug Administration–approved drug to treat delirium, Ely and colleagues are currently conducting a clinical trial to define the role of antipsychotics in the management of delirium in critically ill patients. The study is called the MIND-USA (Modifying the Impact of ICU-Associated Neurologic Dysfunction in the USA) study. It is a multicenter randomized controlled trial comparing the use of haloperidol with ziprasidone. It is scheduled to be completed in February of 2018.

The PAD Bundle and ABCDEF Bundle provide a framework for facilitating implementation of the guidelines. Widespread implementation of either bundle is likely to result in large-scale improvements in ICU patient outcomes. Many resources are available to help with implementation. The guidelines and their tools are endorsed by the American Association of Critical Care Nursing.[42–44] Pun and colleagues[45] published an article presenting 10 key points with strategies to facilitate implementation. The Vanderbilt University Web site offers unrestricted access of materials for use with patient care and provider education.[39] If widely adopted, these guidelines have the potential to broadly transform the care of critically ill patients. These guidelines have the potential to lead to significant improvements in patient outcomes, such as improved pain management, shortened duration of mechanical ventilation, a reduced incidence of delirium, and a significant reduction in costs.[46]

REFERENCES

1. Kollef MH, Levy NT, Ahrens TS, et al. The use of continuous IV sedation is associated with prolongation of mechanical ventilation. Chest 1996;114:541–8.
2. Rello J, Diaz E, Rogue M, et al. Risk factors for developing pneumonia with 48 hours of intubation. Am J Respir Crit Care Med 1999;159(6):1742–6.
3. Kress JP, Pohlman AS, O'Connor MF, et al. Daily interruption of sedative infusions in critically ill patients undergoing mechanical ventilation. N Engl J Med 2000; 342(20):1471–7.
4. Riker RR, Picard JT, Fraser GL. Prospective evaluation of the Sedation-Agitation Scale (SAS) for adult critically ill patients. Crit Care Med 1999;27:1325–9.
5. Sessler CN, Gosnell MS, Grap MJ, et al. The Richmond Agitation-Sedation Scale (RASS): validity and reliability in adult intensive care unit patients. Am J Respir Crit Care Med 2002;166:1338–44.
6. Weisbrodt L, McKinley S, Marshall AP, et al. Daily interruption of sedation in patients receiving mechanical ventilation. Am J Crit Care 2011;20(4):e90–8.
7. Mendez MP, Lazar MH, DiGiovine B, et al. Dedicated multidisciplinary ventilator bundle team and compliance with sedation vacation. Am J Crit Care 2013;22(1): 54–60.
8. Barr J, Fraser GL, Puntillo K, et al. American College of Critical Care Medicine. Clinical practice guidelines for the management of pain, agitation and delirium in adult patients in the intensive care unit. Crit Care Med 2013;41(1):263–306.
9. Jacobi J, Fraser GL, Coursin DB, et al. Clinical practice guidelines for the sustained use of sedatives and analgesics in the critically ill adult. Crit Care Med 2002;30:119–41.
10. Davidson JE, Winkelman C, Gelinas C, et al. Pain, agitation and delirium guidelines: nurses' involvement in development and implementation. Crit Care Nurse 2015;35(3):17–32.
11. Puntillo KA, White C, Morris C, et al. Patients' perceptions and responses to procedural pain: results from Thunder Project II. Am J Crit Care 2001;10(4):238–51.
12. Shannon K, Bucknall T. Pain assessment in critical care: what have we learnt from research? Intensive Crit Care Nurs 2003;19:154–62.
13. Puntillo K, Weiss SJ. Pain: its mediators and associated morbidity in critically ill cardiovascular surgical patients. Nurs Res 1994;43:31–6.
14. Chanques G, Viel E, Constantin JM, et al. The measurement of pain in intensive care unit: comparison of 5 self-report intensity scales. Pain 2010;151(3):711–21.

15. Ahlers SJ, van Gulik L, van der Veen AM, et al. Comparison of different pain scoring systems in critically ill patients in a general intensive care unit. Crit Care 2008;12(1):R15.
16. Chanques G, Jaber S, Barbote E, et al. Impact of systematic evaluation of pain and agitation in an intensive care unit. Crit Care Med 2006;34:1691–9.
17. Herr K, Coyne PJ, McCaffery M, et al. Pain assessment in the patient unable to self-report: position statement with clinical practice recommendations. Pain Manag Nurs 2011;12(4):230–50.
18. Pasero C, McCaffery M. Pain assessment and pharmacologic management. St Louis (MO): Mosby; 2011.
19. Payen J, Bru O, Bosson J, et al. Assessing pain in critically ill sedated pts by using a behavioral pain scale. Crit Care Med 2001;29(12):2258–63.
20. Gelinas C, Fillion L, Puntillo KA, et al. Validation of the critical care pain observation tool in adult patients. Am J Crit Care 2006;15(4):420–7.
21. Grap MJ, Munro CL, Wetzel PA, et al. Sedation in adults receiving mechanical ventilation: physiological and comfort outcomes. Am J Crit Care 2012;21(3): e53–64.
22. Ely EW, Baker AM, Dunagan DP, et al. Effect on the duration of mechanical ventilation of identifying patients capable of breathing spontaneously. N Engl J Med 1996;335:1864–9.
23. Girard TD, Kress JP, Fuchs BD, et al. Efficacy and safety of a paired sedation and ventilator weaning protocol for mechanically ventilated patients in intensive care (Awakening and Breathing Controlled trial): a randomised controlled trial. Lancet 2008;371(9607):126–34.
24. O'Connor M, Bucknall T, Manias E. A critical review of daily sedation interruption in the ICU. J Clin Nurs 2009;18(9):1239–49.
25. Riker RR, Shehai Y, Bokesch PM, et al. Dexmedetomidine vs midazolam for sedation of critically ill patients: a randomized trial. The SEDCOM (safety and efficacy of dexmedetomidine compared with midazolam) study group. JAMA 2009; 301(5):489–99.
26. Schweickert WD, Pohlman MC, Pohlman AS, et al. Early physical and occupational therapy in mechanically ventilated, critically ill patients: a randomised controlled trial. Lancet 2009;373(9678):1874–82.
27. Vollman K. Progressive mobility in the critically ill: introduction to progressive mobility. Crit Care Nurse 2010;30(2):S3–55.
28. American Psychiatric Association. Diagnostic and statistical manual of mental disorders (DSM-IV-TR). Washington, DC: American Psychiatric Association; 2000. p. 143.
29. Ely EW, Shintani A, Truman B, et al. Delirium as a predictor of mortality in mechanically ventilated patients in the intensive care unit. JAMA 2004;291:1753–62.
30. Sona C. Assessing delirium in the intensive care unit. Crit Care Nurse 2009;2: 103–5.
31. Pandharipande PP, Girard TK, Jackson JC, et al. Long-term cognitive impairment after critical illness. N Engl J Med 2013;369:1306–16.
32. Girard TD, Jackson JC, Pandharipande PP, et al. Delirium as a predictor of long-term cognitive impairment in survivors of critical illness. Crit Care Med 2010; 38(7):1513–20.
33. Ely EW, Inouye SK, Bernard GR, et al. Delirium in mechanically ventilated patients: validity and reliability of the confusion assessment method for the intensive care unit. JAMA 2001;286(21):2703–10.
34. Balas MC, Rice M, Chaperon C, et al. Management of delirium in critically ill older adults. Crit Care Nurse 2012;32(4):15–26.

35. Ely EW, Siegel MD, Inouye S, et al. Delirium in the intensive care unit: an under-recognized syndrome of organ dysfunction. Semin Respir Crit Care Med 2001;22: 115–26.

36. Inouye SK, van Dyck CH, Alessi CA, et al. Clarifying confusion: the confusion assessment method. A new method for detection of delirium. Ann Intern Med 1990;113(12):941–8.

37. Bergeron N, Dubois MJ, Dumont M, et al. Intensive care delirium screening checklist: evaluation of a new screening tool. Intensive Care Med 2001;27(5): 859–64.

38. Boehm L, Okahashi J. Measuring success of the ABCDE bundle: dare to make a difference in patient care. Boston (MA): American Association of Critical Care Nurse (AACN) National Teaching Institute; 2013.

39. ICU Delirium and Cognitive Impairment Study Group of Vanderbilt University Medical Center. Available at: www.icudelirium.org. Accessed November 6, 2015.

40. Balas M, Vasilevskis E, Burke W, et al. Critical care nurses' role in implementing the ABCDE Bundle into practice. Crit Care Nurse 2012;32(2):35–8, 40–8.

41. Rivosecchi RM, Smithburger PL, Svec S, et al. Nonpharmacological interventions to prevent delirium: AN evidence-based systematic review. Crit Care Nurse 2015; 35(1):39–51.

42. American Association of Critical Care Nurses (AACN) Practice Alert: Assessing pain in the critically ill adult. Amer Assoc Crit Care Nurses 2013.

43. Bell L. American Association of Critical Care Nurses (AACN) Practice Alert: Delirium assessment and management. Amer Assoc Crit Care Nurses 2011.

44. American Association of Critical Care Nurses. AACN PEARL (Practice, Evidence, Application, Resources and Leadership): Implementation of the ABCDE Bundle, 2012.

45. Pun BT, Balas MC, Davidson J. Implementing the 2013 PAD guidelines: top ten points to consider. Semin Respir Crit Care Med 2013;34:223–35.

46. Barr J, Pandharipande PP. The pain, agitation and delirium care bundle: synergistic benefits of implementing the 2013 pain, agitation and delirium guidelines in an integrated and interdisciplinary fashion. Crit Care Med 2013;41(9 Suppl 1):S99–115.

Patient Safety
Identifying and Managing Complications of Mechanical Ventilation

Heather Baid, RN, BSN, PGCHSCE, PGCert, MSc

KEYWORDS

- Ventilator-associated event • Ventilator-associated condition
- Ventilator-associated infection • Ventilator-associated pneumonia
- Acute respiratory distress syndrome • Pulmonary edema • Pleural effusion
- Atelectasis

KEY POINTS

- The umbrella term of ventilator-associated events (VAEs) is associated with infectious and noninfectious causes of mechanical ventilation complications.
- VAEs can be classified as ventilator-associated conditions (VACs), ventilator-associated infections (IVACs), or ventilator-associated pneumonia.
- Common VAEs in critical care are discussed according to the current literature base for each including ventilator-associated pneumonia, acute respiratory distress syndrome, pulmonary edema, pleural effusion, and atelectasis.

INTRODUCTION

Mechanical ventilation is an essential intervention provided by critical care services, although there are several potential complications that result from being mechanically ventilated. These ventilator-associated events (VAEs) can be infectious or noninfectious in nature as indicated in **Table 1**. It is important to identify the type and cause of a VAE to help plan clinical management, which is then specifically aimed at treating the source of the mechanical ventilation problem. A thorough understanding of how different VAEs arise will also enable critical care nurses to underpin their clinical practice with measures to prevent complications of mechanical ventilation from occurring. Essential preventative strategies include avoiding intubation where possible, keeping the duration of mechanical ventilation to a minimum, and actively targeting the most common causes of VAEs.[1]

The purpose of this article is to critically discuss the prevention, identification, and management of the major complications of mechanical ventilation within the context of critical care nursing practice. Current research and gaps in the evidence base for

School of Health Sciences, University of Brighton, Westlain House, Village Way, Falmer Campus, Brighton BN1 9PH, UK
E-mail address: H.Baid@brighton.ac.uk

Crit Care Nurs Clin N Am 28 (2016) 451–462
http://dx.doi.org/10.1016/j.cnc.2016.07.005
0899-5885/16/Crown Copyright © 2016 Published by Elsevier Inc. All rights reserved.
ccnursing.theclinics.com

Table 1 Ventilator-associated events	
Infectious	**Noninfectious**
Pneumonia	ARDS
	Pulmonary edema
	Pleural effusion
	Atelectasis

each topic will be highlighted throughout, and **Table 2** provides a summary of the nursing assessment findings and management associated with each complication.

VENTILATOR-ASSOCIATED PNEUMONIA

Ventilator-associated pneumonia (VAP) lacks a universal, internationally agreed definition as now exists for other common conditions in critical care such as sepsis,[2] acute coronary syndromes,[3] and acute respiratory distress syndrome.[4] The subjective nature of traditional VAP diagnosis methods, along with a high degree of inter-rater variability and inaccuracy, has meant many patients who previously met VAP diagnostic criteria did not actually have pneumonia.[5]

Magill and colleagues[6] address these issues with a new framework for the surveillance of VAEs.

Ventilator-associated condition (VAC) is defined as baseline of at least 2 days of stability with decreasing daily Fio_2 and positive end–expiratory pressure (PEEP) requirements, as well as subsequent deteriorating hypoxemia sustained for at least ≥ 2 days with daily Fio_2 increase of at least 0.20 or PEEP increase of at least 3 cm H_2O from the baseline period.

Ventilator-associated infection (IVAC) is defined as the VAC points described previously, as well as altered temperature (<36°C or 38°C) or leukocytes ($\leq$4000 cells/mm^3 or $\geq$12,000 cells/mm^3) and new antimicrobial(s) introduced and administered for $\geq$4 days.

VAP can be divided into 2 categories:

Possible VAP—quantitatively purulent secretions or positive culture from respiratory tract
Probable VAP—quantitatively purulent secretions and positive culture from respiratory tract or positive results from pleural fluid culture, lung histopathology, or other specific diagnostic tests[7]

Although this new perspective on defining and measuring VAP is a more objective process compared with previous practice, several things need to be considered:

- The publication by Magill and colleagues[6] stems from a VAP working group convened by the US Centers for Disease Control and Prevention[7] and included representatives from US organizations; other countries need to evaluate whether these recommendations are relevant to their own health care practice.
- The new definitions are not proposed for use in the clinical management of patients but aim to be for surveillance monitoring.
- Research is still needed on whether this new surveillance format is: valid and reliable in being linked to associated clinical outcomes, able to identify all types of pneumonia, and capable of improving VAP prevention and early detection in critical care units.[8]

Table 2
Ventilator-associated events: nursing assessment findings and actions

Type of VAC	Nursing Assessment Findings Associated with the VAC	Nursing Interventions to Act Upon the VAC
VAP	• Risk factors: aspiration during intubation, multiple intubations, immune compromised, COPD, ARDS, chronic disease, recent hospitalization • High or low temperature • Sputum—large amounts, thick and abnormal color and consistency (thick, yellow, green, purulent) • Lung percussion—dullness over area of likely infection • Lung auscultation—crackles, bronchial breath sound to area of likely infection (where vesicular sounds would be expected) • High or low leukocytes and other inflammatory markers (c-reactive protein [CRP], procalcitonin)	• Send sputum sample to laboratory and consider whether blood cultures, urine, and other samples also indicated • Suction as required • Nebulizers as required • Monitor and document color, consistency, and quantity of sputum • Administer anti-microbial agents as prescribed • Liaise with critical care doctor and pharmacist with updates on patient status to contribute to antimicrobial stewardship while prescriptions are being reviewed • Monitor for signs of sepsis and follow sepsis care bundles if indicated
ARDS	• Risk factors: sepsis, ventilator-induced lung injury, aspiration, pneumonia, toxic inhalation, near drowning, trauma, hypothermia, massive transfusion, pancreatitis • Low Pao_2:Fio_2 ratio • Chest expansion—reduced if low tidal volumes • Lung percussion—dullness to areas of abnormality • Lung auscultation—diminished breath sounds likely to lower lung fields, fine crackles if pulmonary edema present	• Treatment for underlying cause • Protective lung strategies: tidal volumes 6–8 mL/kg, Fio_2-guided PEEP, plateau pressure <30 cm H_2O • Monitor for infection and treat accordingly • Monitor for pleural effusion and treat accordingly • Conservative fluid management and negative fluid balance • Diuretics and renal replacement therapy as indicated • Oxygenation strategies—inverse I:E ratio, APRV mode, proning, extracorporeal membrane oxygenation • Severe ARDS—early use neuromuscular blocking agent ≤48 h of onset)
Pulmonary edema	• Risk factors: heart failure, ARDS, renal dysfunction, lung injury • Sputum—large amounts and abnormal color and consistency (pink, frothy) • May also have signs of peripheral edema • Lung percussion—dullness to areas of likely pulmonary edema • Lung auscultation—fine crackles (wet sounding) to areas of likely pulmonary edema	• Upright positioning • Diuretics • PEEP • Renal replacement therapy as indicated • Hemodynamic monitoring • Inotropes/intra-aortic balloon pump as indicated for cardiogenic shock

(continued on next page)

Type of VAC	Nursing Assessment Findings Associated with the VAC	Nursing Interventions to Act Upon the VAC

Table 2
(*continued*)

Type of VAC	Nursing Assessment Findings Associated with the VAC	Nursing Interventions to Act Upon the VAC
Pleural effusion	• Risk factors: fluid overload, pneumonia, ARDS, atelectasis heart failure, renal dysfunction, liver failure, sepsis, massive transfusion • Chest expansion—reduced to lower thorax (unilateral if one, bilateral if both lungs have an effusion) • Lung percussion—dullness to area of likely effusion • Lung auscultation—absent sound over area of likely effusion	• Upright positioning • Monitoring for deterioration in tidal volume and respiratory status if asymptomatic effusion • Diuretics • Drainage • Monitor color and amount of pleural fluid if drained • Send pleural fluid sample to laboratory • PEEP • If large effusion, monitor for signs of hemodynamic compromise
Atelectasis	• Risk factors: low tidal volumes, high Fio_2, mucous plugging, postoperative, abdominal/thoracic pain, obesity • Chest expansion—reduced to area of likely atelectasis • Lung percussion—dullness to area of likely atelectasis • Lung auscultation—fine crackles (dry sounding) to area of likely atelectasis or diminished sounds if a large region affected	• Upright positioning • Tidal volumes 6–8 mL/kg • PEEP • Pain management • Physiotherapy • Mobility if possible • Suctioning as required
Pneumothorax	• Risk factors: high plateau pressures, high PEEP, ARDS, asthma, COPD, iatrogenic procedures (central line, tracheostomy, surgery to thorax or lower neck) • Tracheal deviation away from affected lung • Chest expansion—unilateral • Lung percussion—hyperresonance over affected lung • Lung auscultation—absent breath sounds over affected lung	• Monitor for signs of respiratory deterioration if not being actively treated • Chest drain as required—monitor for cessation of air bubbling in drain management system • Monitor tidal volumes and plateau pressure

If any of these VACs are clinically significant, there will be signs of acute respiratory failure due to poor gas exchange as seen with low SaO_2, low Pao_2, high $Paco_2$, and/or increased respiratory rate and effort if there are spontaneous breaths. Nursing actions related to the ventilator can then be tailored to improve the specific gas exchange needs of that patient at the time of the nursing assessment.

The updated terminology related to VAP[6] does however have the benefit of encouraging practitioners to differentiate infectious from non-infectious causes of complications of mechanical ventilation. The promotion of a robust, standardized approach to identifying VAP can also help with the comparison of infection rates between critical care units which can then lead to the improvement for how VAP is prevented or clinically managed once it occurs. VAP is the most frequent and significant infection related VAC and preventative strategies are therefore of utmost importance. Critical care nurses typically follow a clustered approach for VAP prevention (see **Table 3** for an example of a VAP care bundle).

Table 3
Care bundle for ventilator-associated pneumonia prevention[9,10]

Care Bundle Element	Rationale
Head of bed elevation (30°–45°)	Prevention of oropharyngeal and gastric content aspiration[11]
Spontaneous awakening trial + spontaneous breathing trial	Promotion and evaluation of readiness to wean, and extubate, and for removal of mechanical ventilation[12]
Subglottic secretion drainage plus tube cuff pressure >20 cm H_2O	Prevention of section aspiration from above the oral endotracheal tube cuff[13]
Change ventilator tubing and suction systems only when clinically indicated	Frequent changes of allow greater opportunity for introduction of pathogens to the patient[14]

Data from Refs.[9–14]

More recent meta-analyses[15,16] and a randomized control trial[17] concluded that subglottic secretion drainage significantly reduced VAP occurrence but did not reduce time spent on the ventilator, intensive care or hospital length of stay, VAEs, mortality, or antibiotic use. This then highlights there remains an ongoing debate and need for further research about the clinical effectiveness of subglottic secretion drainage.

There are additional interventions that have been widely used within VAP care bundles but a lack of evidence and conflicting research studies have resulted in removal of the element or the recommendation to use with caution. One such change, following a recent meta-analysis[18] and other research,[19] has been to no longer recommend oral chlorhexidine except for cardiac surgery intensive care patients. The British National Institute for Clinical Excellence[20] has formally withdrawn previous guidance on administering oral chlorhexidine, because the current evidence base no longer supports this and due to the potential risks of harm. Oral care measures, such as tooth brushing, oral irrigation, oropharyngeal suctioning, and tongue cleaning, however, are still conducted for patient comfort, dental hygiene, and likely VAP prevention. However, much of the research on this type of mouth care has been done in combination or comparison with chlorhexidine, and further studies on best practice for oral hygiene care are still needed.[21]

The silver-coated endotracheal tube is another intervention with limited evidence but some indication it may be helpful in preventing VAP.[22] Selective decontamination of the digestive tract (SDD) has also shown the ability to reduce VAP and mortality, but concern about antibiotic resistance has created controversy and deterred widespread adoption of SDD.[23,24] Further research may provide a clearer consensus on the routine use of SDD such as from the upcoming SuDDICU randomized control trial.[25] Additionally, more research is needed in relation to gastrointestinal stress ulcer prophylaxis (SUP) because of conflicting evidence on whether SUP influences VAP rates (increasing or decreasing VAP depending on whether a proton pump inhibitor or H_2 antagonist is given), along with a possible increased risk of *Clostridium difficile* infection with SUP use.[26,27] SUP continues to be widely used because of gastrointestinal bleeding being a potential complication of mechanically ventilated patients, although the move toward early enteral feeding when possible and the results of future bigger clinical trials may challenge this practice in the future.

There are other interventions that can be included in a more generalized approach to care bundles aimed at preventing all types of VAEs including noninfectious VACs. However, there is potential for actions to simultaneously overlap with VAP prevention by leading to earlier liberation from mechanical ventilation. Therefore, in addition to the actions listed in **Table 3**, the following interventions are recommended with the intention of directly or indirectly preventing VAP and helping to prevent other potential complications of mechanical ventilation[1,28–30]:

- Minimize sedation and avoid benzodiazepines when possible
- Early mobility and ambulation when possible
- Lung-protective strategies
- Conservative fluid management
- Conservative transfusion of blood products
- Deep venous thrombosis prophylaxis
- Hand hygiene and personal protective equipment when clinically indicated
- Avoid nonessential tracheal suctioning
- Avoid gastric overdistension

If VAP is suspected, nurses should ensure a sputum sample has been sent to the laboratory and highlight the suspicious clinical findings to the member of the critical care team responsible for deciding whether antibiotics are indicated. Once antibiotics have been given for 72 hours,[31] nurses can contribute to discussions about when to discontinue antibiotics and/or if other more selective antimicrobial agents are required, thereby promoting the appropriate use of antimicrobial drugs. Antimicrobial stewardship and an overall reduction in antibiotic consumption through VAE prevention programs may be identified as quality indicators for critical care unit performance.[32] It is thus important for nurses to have an awareness of their role in drug therapy for infections.

Finally, nurses should be attentive to signs of sepsis and continually monitor whether the VAP has triggered a septic episode. The Quick Sequential Organ Failure Assessment (qSOFA) screening tool highlights that sepsis should be considered if at least 2 out of these 3 points are present: hypotension, altered mental status, and tachypnea.[2] However, with a sedated patient on a mandatory mode of ventilation, the qSOFA score may not be relevant, and a change from baseline of 2 or more points using the total SOFA score would be a more accurate screening method.[2] Management of sepsis should then follow the sepsis care bundles, which in addition to blood cultures and antibiotics, should include monitoring lactate, crystalloid infusion for hypotension, and vasopressors to maintain mean arterial pressure of at least 65 mm Hg.[33]

ACUTE RESPIRATORY DISTRESS SYNDROME

Acute respiratory distress syndrome (ARDS) occurs when diffuse lung injury activates extensive inflammation throughout the lungs, disrupting the alveolar–capillary membrane and resulting in significantly impaired gas exchange. As a syndrome, ARDS has a collection of associated clinical findings, with the Berlin definition of ARDS[4] defining these as

- Presentation less than a week before a known insult, or new or deteriorating respiratory status
- Chest radiograph–bilateral opacities not attributable to effusions, lobar/lung collapse, or nodules
- Noncardiogenic pulmonary edema
- With a minimum continuous positive airway pressure (CPAP) or PEEP level of 5 cm H_2O, oxygenation status
  - Mild ARDS—Pao_2:Fio_2 201 to 300 mm Hg ($\leq$39.9 kPa).
  - Moderate ARDS—Pao_2:Fio_2 101 to 200 mm Hg ($\leq$26.6 kPa).
  - Severe ARDS—Pao_2:Fio_2 no more than 100 mm Hg ($\leq$13.3 kPa).

The Large Observational Study to Understand the Global Impact of Severe Acute Respiratory Failure (LUNG SAFE) study took place in 459 intensive care units from 50 countries ($n = 29,144$) and revealed the period prevalence of ARDS was 10.4% of intensive care admissions and 23.4% of patients who were mechanically ventilated.[34] This study also indicated a hospital mortality of 34.9% for mild ARDS, 40.3% for moderate ARDS, and 46.1% for patients with severe ARDS.

There is an overlap between nursing interventions to prevent and act upon ARDS, particularly with the ventilation settings and monitoring. Protective lung strategies involve an open lung perspective to mechanical ventilation underpinned by a high PEEP, low tidal volume approach. In practical terms, this means ensuring tidal volumes fall between 6 and 8 mL/kg; the plateau pressure remains less than 30 cm H_2O; and relatively high amounts of PEEP guided by the Fio_2 level are used to recruit alveoli. Despite permissive hypoxemia not being supported by research,[35,36] it is common practice to not aim for normal oxygenation values, and instead, to accept relatively low SaO_2 and Pao_2 values. It is unclear whether permissive hypoxemia is beneficial but avoiding hyperoxemia is thought to be likely warranted.[37]

Permissive hypercapnia is also typically used with ARDS patients (allowing a higher than normal $Paco_2$ as long as the pH is >7.25), although a recent meta-analysis[38] identifies that permissive hypercapnia along with recruitment maneuvers and low airway pressures are the specific ventilation strategies with the highest mortality. This meta-analysis of 36 randomized control trials ($n = 6685$ patients)[38] concluded that these strategies are associated with a lower mortality:

- Higher tidal volumes plus Fio_2 guided lower PEEP.
- Pressure-controlled ventilation plus Fio_2 guided lower PEEP.
- Lower tidal volumes plus Fio_2 guided lower PEEP and prone positioning.

The meta-analysis[39] also suggests that the strategies that show potential for being the optimal method of ventilating ARDS patients are

- Lower tidal volumes plus FiO_2-guided higher PEEP plus prone positioning ventilation
- Lower tidal volumes plus pressure-volume (P–V) static curve-guided individual PEEP

There is insufficient research currently to indicate whether a pressure-controlled or volume-controlled mode is advantageous compared with the other for ARDS patients.[40] Airway pressure release ventilation (APRV) mode shows potential, because it maximizes alveolar recruitment, allows for reduced sedation and spontaneous breathing, and increases ventilation of dependent regions; however, despite improvement in oxygenation while used as a rescue therapy, there is no research yet to show APRV improves other outcomes.[41] Other therapies with recent research to support them as interventions for ARDS include early use of proning ($\leq$48 hours after severe ARDS onset) for prolonged periods (16 hours sessions),[42] neuromuscular blockade ($\leq$48 hours after severe ARDS onset),[43] and maintaining a negative fluid balance.[44] If refractory hypoxemia remains despite other efforts, extracorporeal membrane oxygenation (ECMO) is then indicated.[45]

PULMONARY EDEMA

A large number of VAEs (20%–40%) are related to fluid overload in some way, with mechanical ventilation being indirectly involved in the development of this excessive fluid in the lungs.[1] The nursing assessment and management of fluid status are essential aspects of caring for a mechanically ventilated patients, because a positive fluid balance is an independent risk factor for VAEs including VAP and ARDS.[46] Conservative fluid management can significantly improve weaning[47] and decrease VAEs,[1] and excessive fluid overload increases morbidity and mortality of ventilated patients, particularly with septic patients.[1] Fine crackles are definitive for pulmonary edema on auscultation and requires diuresis and/or renal replacement therapy to offload fluid.

PLEURAL EFFUSION

The prevalence of pleural effusions in intensive care is 62%, with common causes being fluid overload, atelectasis, pneumonia, postoperative complications, and malignancy.[48] Mechanical ventilation may therefore be an indirect cause of effusions if contribution to these types of conditions but it can also help with the management with PEEP being used to improve oxygenation and decrease the workload of breathing that was affected by large or bilateral effusions. Pleural effusions can be small and relatively insignificant requiring only monitoring. Pleural effusions present with dullness on percussion and reduced chest expansion and absent breath sounds over an effusion due to lung tissue not being able to expand into that area, typically the lower parts of the lungs. If treatment of pleural effusion is needed, this can include diuretics and drainage of the effusion.

ATELECTASIS

Atelectasis is defined as the collapse of alveoli, and it can affect a small area of the lungs (typically the lower lung fields), a full lobe (lobar atelectasis), or a whole lung. Atelectasis is common with intensive care patients and can be a complication of mechanical ventilation if tidal volumes are low, causing mechanical collapse, or high Fio_2 delivery leads to absorption atelectasis.[49] Postoperative patients are particularly at risk of atelectasis, because the supine position for a long period of perioperative time increases the risk of alveolar collapse. Abdominal or thoracic pain preventing the patient from making much effort with spontaneous breaths is a further consideration while trying to identify a cause of atelectasis. Atelectasis can also be attributed to obesity, mucous plugging, air trapping, pleural effusion, and ARDS.[50]

If the alveoli pop open during inspiration but collapse again on expiration (cyclic atelectasis), fine crackles may be heard on auscultation. A larger area of collapsed alveoli or lobar/lung collapse can result in dullness on percussion and absent breath sounds. PEEP can help to prevent and resolve atelectasis and also reduce the risk of ventilator-induced lung injury if the PEEP helps improve cyclic atelectasis. Physiotherapy, mobilization, sitting up, and ensuring mechanical ventilation settings are used appropriately for sufficient tidal volume and lowest possible Fio_2 are all strategies to address atelectasis.

PNEUMOTHORAX

A pneumothorax is also lung collapse but differs from atelectasis in that it is due to air in the pleural cavity after injury or weak tissue causes the pleura to come away from the chest wall. A pneumothorax can be a complication of mechanical ventilation, particularly when high amounts of PEEP and an inverse ratio are used. Most intensive care patients with a pneumothorax have a pre-existing respiratory condition such as pneumonia, ARDS, or chronic obstructive pulmonary disease (COPD).[51] Clinical findings of a pneumothorax include: tracheal deviation away from the affected lung, reduced chest expansion unilaterally, hyper-resonance on lung percussion, and absent breath sounds on auscultation. A small pneumothorax may resolve on its own; otherwise a chest tube is needed to allow the displaced air to leave the pleural space and for the lung to then reinflate.

SUMMARY

This discussion has focused on 5 common ventilator-associated events that can occur as a direct or indirect complication of mechanical ventilation. Nurses caring for critically ill patients should also consider the influence mechanical ventilation has on other organs besides the lungs such as: airway damage during intubation or tracheostomy insertion; hypotension from changes in intrathoracic pressure leading to secondary hemodynamic compromise, acute kidney injury and liver dysfunction; and impact on cerebral perfusion pressure, which may be of significance for neurologic patients. Assessing and supporting the patient and family member's psychosocial well-being as affected by the mechanical ventilation is also a crucial part of holistic nursing practice. Finally, in addition to technical knowledge and skill, nontechnical skills such as communication, teamwork, and situational awareness are just as important for preventing, identifying, and managing complications of mechanical ventilation. By attending to technical and nontechnical aspects of clinical practice, nurses are then able to provide safe, effective and high quality critical care while nursing mechanically ventilated patients.

REFERENCES

1. Klompas M. Potential strategies to prevent ventilator-associated events. Am J Respir Crit Care Med 2015;192(12):1420–30.
2. Singer M, Deutschman CS, Seymour CW, et al. The Third International Consensus Definitions for Sepsis and Septic Shock (Sepsis-3). JAMA 2016; 315(8):801–10.
3. Thygesen K, Alpert JS, Jaffe AS, et al. Third universal definition of myocardial infarction. Eur Heart J 2012;33(20):2551–67.
4. The ARDS Definition Task Force, Ranieri VM, Rubenfeld GD, Thompson BT, et al. Acute respiratory distress syndrome: the Berlin Definition. JAMA 2012;307(23):2526–33.
5. Klompas M. Complications of mechanical ventilation — The CDC's New Surveillance Paradigm. N Engl J Med 2013;368(16):1472–5.
6. Magill SS, Klompas M, Balk R, et al. Developing a new, national approach to surveillance for ventilator-associated events. Crit Care Med 2013;41(11): 2467–75.
7. Centers for Disease Control and Prevention. Surveillance for ventilator-associated events. 2016. Available at: http://www.cdc.gov/nhsn/acute-care-hospital/vae/index.html. Accessed July 4, 2016.
8. Pugh R, Szakmany T. Ventilator-associated pneumonia surveillance: complex, complicated and still searching for the best tool. Br J Intensive Care 2014; 24(1):20–5.
9. Hellyer TP, Simpson AJ. Ventilator-associated pneumonia. Guidelines for the provision of intensive care services. 2015. p. 102–4. Available at: www.ficm.ac.uk/sites/default/files/GPICS%20-%20Ed.1%20%282015%29_0.pdf. Accessed July 4, 2016.
10. Hellyer TP, Ewan V, Wilson P, et al. The intensive care society recommended bundle of interventions for the prevention of ventilator-associated pneumonia. J Intensive Care Soc 2016;17(3):238–43.

11. Wang L, Li X, Yang Z, et al. Semi-recumbent position versus supine position for the prevention of ventilator-associated pneumonia in adults requiring mechanical ventilation. Cochrane Database Syst Rev 2016;(1):CD009946.

12. Klompas M, Anderson D, Trick W, et al. The preventability of ventilator-associated events. The CDC prevention epicenters wake up and breathe collaborative. Am J Respir Crit Care Med 2015;191(3):292–301.

13. Frost SA, Azeem A, Alexandrou E, et al. Subglottic secretion drainage for preventing ventilator associated pneumonia: a meta-analysis. Aust Crit Care 2013; 26(4):180–8.

14. Rello J, Afonso E, Lisboa T, et al. A care bundle approach for prevention of ventilator-associated pneumonia. Clin Microbiol Infect 2013;19(4):363–9.

15. Damas P, Frippiat F, Ancion A, et al. Prevention of ventilator-associated pneumonia and ventilator-associated conditions. Crit Care Med 2015;43(1):22–30.

16. Roquilly A, Marret E, Abraham E, et al. Pneumonia prevention to decrease mortality in intensive care unit: a systematic review and meta-analysis. Clin Infect Dis 2015;60(1):64–75.

17. Caroff DA, Li L, Muscedere J, et al. Subglottic secretion drainage and objective outcomes. Crit Care Med 2015;44(4):830–40.

18. Klompas M, Speck K, Howell MD, et al. Reappraisal of routine oral care with chlorhexidine gluconate for patients receiving mechanical ventilation. JAMA 2014;174(5):751.

19. Wong T, Schlichting AB, Stoltze AJ, et al. No decrease in early ventilator-associated pneumonia after early use of chlorhexidine. Am J Crit Care 2016; 25(2):173–7.

20. National Institute for Health and Care Excellence. Technical patient safety solutions for ventilator-associated pneumonia in adults. 2016. Available at: https://www.nice.org.uk/guidance/psg2. Accessed July 4, 2016.

21. Shi Z, Xie H, Wang P, et al. Oral hygiene care for critically ill patients to prevent ventilator associated pneumonia. Cochrane Database Syst Rev 2013;(8):CD008367.

22. Tokmaji G, Vermeulen H, Müller MC, et al. Silver coated endotracheal tubes for prevention of ventilator-associated pneumonia in critically ill patients. Cochrane Database Syst Rev 2015;(8):CD009201.

23. Price RJ, Cuthbertson BH. Selective decontamination of the digestive tract and oropharynx: after 30 years of debate is the definitive answer in sight? Curr Opin Crit Care 2016;22(2):161–6.

24. Silvestri L, van Saene HK. Selective decontamination of the digestive tract: an update of the evidence. HSR Proc Intensive Care Cardiovasc Anesth 2012;4(1):21–9.

25. Cuthbertson B, Cook D, Bellingan G. SuDDICU—Selective decontamination of the digestive track in the ICU. 2016. Available at: http://www.ccctg.ca/Programs/SuDDICU-study.aspx. Accessed July 4, 2016.

26. Fohl AL, Regal RE. Proton pump inhibitor-associated pneumonia: not a breath of fresh air after all. World J Gastrointest Pharmacol Ther 2011;2(3):17–26.

27. Krag M, Perner A, Wetterslev J, et al. Stress ulcer prophylaxis in the intensive care unit: an international survey of 97 units in 11 countries. Acta Anaesthesiol Scand 2015;59(5):576–85.

28. Raoof S, Baumann MH. Ventilator-associated events: the new definition. Am J Crit Care 2014;23(1):7–9.

29. Sedwick MB, Lance-Smith M, Reeder SJ, et al. Using evidence-based practice to prevent ventilator-associated pneumonia. Crit Care Nurse 2012;32(4):41–51.

30. Speck K, Rawat N, Weiner NC, et al. A systematic approach for developing a ventilator-associated pneumonia prevention bundle. Am J Infect Control 2016; 44(6):652–6.

31. Nair GB, Niederman MS. Ventilator-associated pneumonia: present understanding and ongoing debates. Intensive Care Med 2015;41(1):34–48.

32. Bouadma L, Sonneville R, Garrouste-Orgeas M, et al. Ventilator-associated events: prevalence, outcome, and relationship with ventilator-associated pneumonia. Crit Care Med 2015;43(9):1798–806.

33. Surviving Sepsis Campaign. Surviving Sepsis Campaign bundles. 2015. Available at: http://www.survivingsepsis.org/Bundles/Pages/default.aspx. Accessed July 4, 2016.

34. Bellani G, Laffey JG, Pham T, et al. Epidemiology, patterns of care, and mortality for patients with acute respiratory distress syndrome in intensive care units in 50 countries. JAMA 2016;315(8):788.

35. Martin DS, Grocott MP. Oxygen therapy in critical illness: precise control of arterial oxygenation and permissive hypoxemia. Crit Care Med 2013;41(2):423–32.

36. Gilbert-Kawai ET, Mitchell K, Martin D, et al. Permissive hypoxaemia versus normoxaemia for mechanically ventilated critically ill patients. Cochrane Database Syst Rev 2014;(1):CD009931.

37. González S. Permissive hypoxemia versus normoxemia for critically ill patients receiving mechanical ventilation. Crit Care Nurse 2015;35(2):80–1.

38. Wang C, Wang X, Chi C, et al. Lung ventilation strategies for acute respiratory distress syndrome: a systematic review and network meta-analysis. Sci Rep 2016;6:22855.

39. Chao YC, Chen Y, Wang KK, et al. Removal of oral secretion prior to position change can reduce the incidence of ventilator-associated pneumonia for adult ICU patients: a clinical controlled trial study. J Clin Nurs 2009;18(1):22–8.

40. Chacko B, Peter JV, Tharyan P, et al. Pressure-controlled versus volume-controlled ventilation for acute respiratory failure due to acute lung injury (ALI) or acute respiratory distress syndrome (ARDS). Cochrane Database Syst Rev 2015;(1):CD008807.

41. Daoud EG, Farag HL, Chatburn RL. Airway pressure release ventilation: what do we know? Respir Care 2012;57(2):282–92.

42. Guérin C, Reignier J, Richard JC, et al. Prone positioning in severe acute respiratory distress syndrome. N Engl J Med 2013;368(23):2159–68.

43. Alhazzani W, Alshahrani M, Jaeschke R, et al. Neuromuscular blocking agents in acute respiratory distress syndrome: a systematic review and meta-analysis of randomized controlled trials. Crit Care 2013;17(2):1.

44. Bein T, Grasso S, Moerer O, et al. The standard of care of patients with ARDS: ventilatory settings and rescue therapies for refractory hypoxemia. Intensive Care Med 2016;42(5):699–711.

45. Aokage T, Palmér K, Ichiba S, et al. Extracorporeal membrane oxygenation for acute respiratory distress syndrome. J Intensive Care 2015;3(1):1.

46. Lewis SC, Li L, Murphy MV, et al. Risk factors for ventilator-associated events: a case-control multivariable analysis. Crit Care Med 2014;42(8):1839.

47. Dessap AM, Katsahian S, Roche-Campo F, et al. Ventilator-associated pneumonia during weaning from mechanical ventilation: role of fluid management. Chest 2014;146(1):58–65.

48. Maslove DM, Chen BT, Wang H, et al. The diagnosis and management of pleural effusions in the ICU. J Intensive Care Med 2013;28(1):24–36.

49. Satoshi S, Eastwood GM, Goodwin MD, et al. Atelectasis and mechanical ventilation mode during conservative oxygen therapy: a before-and-after study. J Crit Care 2015;30(6):1232–7.
50. Ray K, Bodenham A, Paramasivam E. Pulmonary atelectasis in anaesthesia and critical care. Con Ed Anaesth Crit Care Pain 2014;14(5):236–45.
51. Hsu CW, Sun SF. Iatrogenic pneumothorax related to mechanical ventilation. World J Crit Care Med 2014;3(1):8.

Special Considerations in the Nursing Care of Mechanically Ventilated Children

CrossMark

Karen Dryden-Palmer, RN, MSN[a],*, Jason Macartney, RRT[b],
Leanne Davidson, RRT[c], Faiza Syed, RRT[d],
Cathy Daniels, RN(EC), MS, NP-Paediatrics[d], Shaindy Alexander, BA, CCLS[e]

KEYWORDS

- Children • Mechanical ventilation • Critical care • Nursing • Noninvasive ventilation
- Developmental support • Long-term ventilation

KEY POINTS

- A key lung protective strategy for mechanical ventilation of children has been to limit tidal volume exposure; however, measuring tidal volume in children can be challenging and difficult to interpret.
- The shift toward use of noninvasive ventilation in critically ill children has exposed new challenges for critical care nurses. Limited availability of size-appropriate technology and developmental factors are important considerations for providing noninvasive ventilation to children.
- Children requiring long-term ventilation are often cared for in critical care environments and the attention of critical care nurses to the long-term implications of ventilation dependence is key in providing best practice.
- Attention to the cognitive, social, and emotional needs of ventilated children can minimize the negative impacts of the critical care experience and improve outcomes for the child and family.

Disclosure: The authors have nothing to disclose.
[a] Paediatric Critical Care Unit, The Hospital for Sick Children, Room 2898, 555 University Avenue, Toronto, Ontario M5G 1X8, Canada; [b] Respiratory Therapy, Paediatric Critical Care Unit, Paediatric Intensive Care Unit, The Hospital for Sick Children, Room 2849, 555 University Avenue, Toronto, Ontario M5G 1X8, Canada; [c] Respiratory Therapy, Cardiac Critical Care Unit, The Hospital for Sick Children, Room 2849, 555 University Avenue, Toronto, Ontario M5G 1X8, Canada; [d] Long-term Ventilation Program, Division of Respiratory Medicine, The Hospital for Sick Children, 4th Floor Hill Wing, 555 University Avenue, Toronto, Ontario M5G 1X8, Canada; [e] Child Life Department, The Hospital for Sick Children, 555 University Avenue, Toronto, Ontario M5G 1X8, Canada
* Corresponding author.
E-mail address: karen.dryden-palmer@sickkids.ca

Crit Care Nurs Clin N Am 28 (2016) 463–475
http://dx.doi.org/10.1016/j.cnc.2016.07.006
0899-5885/16/Crown Copyright © 2016 Published by Elsevier Inc. All rights reserved.
ccnursing.theclinics.com

INTRODUCTION

Mechanical ventilation is an essential lifesaving technology that is often required to treat and to support the recovery of critically ill children.[1,2] Mechanical ventilation with positive pressure delivered both invasively and noninvasively supports the treatment of acute critical illness and ongoing chronic acute disease in children with increasing frequency.[3] Actual or potential respiratory failure arising from either acute or chronic disease processes and their associated treatments can be frightening and highly stressful experiences for children and for their families. Understanding the unique needs of the maturing physiology of the child; designing supportive care that is sensitive to the changing developmental, social, and emotional needs of the child; and delivering care that is aligned with the principles of family-centered care is paramount to ensuring best outcomes for these vulnerable patients. This article describes unique considerations in providing ventilation support for children. It addresses, through a multidisciplinary lens, pediatric considerations for invasive and noninvasive ventilation, the unique needs of long-term ventilated children and their families in critical care, and discusses approaches to meeting the holistic needs of critically ill ventilated children and families.

INVASIVE VENTILATION CONSIDERATIONS

Invasive mechanical ventilation in the intensive care setting is a supportive therapy that is provided to a large number of critically ill children.[3] Although the ventilator is used to support children through recovery, the specific strategies used by clinicians to provide mechanical ventilation therapy to children may lead to complications of ventilator-induced lung injury.[4] Children are at risk for hyperinflation and resulting barotrauma because of physiologic and technological challenges related to their small size, chest wall compliance, and the limitations of ventilator technology.[5] Caregivers must understand not only the basic principles of mechanical ventilation but also the potential contributors to complications for these in children in order to provide safe and effective ventilation support.

Much of the evidence available to guide lung protective ventilation strategies for children has been founded on the adult patient experience. This body of information and clinical experience has informed the care of pediatric patients receiving mechanical ventilation in the absence of the robust evaluation of practices specific to critically ill children.[6] The unique circumstances encountered in the pediatric population challenge critical care nurses and create complexities in the application of these practices to deliver and monitor mechanical ventilation safely in this population. One of the most significant challenges is the measurement and targeting of appropriate tidal volumes in pediatric patients.

Critically ill children's lungs can be easily overdistended and are vulnerable to ventilator-induced lung injury. Ventilation for children has predominantly used pressure-targeted breaths to set appropriate mechanical ventilation parameters.[7] This method of providing mechanical breaths exposes the lung to a controlled pressure level during inspiration.

This approach provides tidal volume delivery that depends on and responds to the physical characteristics of the lung; mainly pulmonary compliance and airway resistance. Ventilation pressures are then adapted to the individual children's needs based on subjective measures such as the observed chest movement and the child's work of breathing.

Technology to measure tidal volumes during mechanical ventilation of infants and small children was not available until the 1990s and the advent of microprocessor controlled ventilators. Newer generations of mechanical ventilators can be configured to deliver preset tidal volumes to small infants and children (volume controlled ventilation). Although technology is improving, accurate evaluation of tidal volumes for children remains problematic. Critical care nurses must account for several important limiting factors in interpreting the volume ventilation needs of children. Tidal volume measurements can be affected by the type of and size of endotracheal tube. Smaller diameter endotracheal tubes available for children have until recently been uncuffed. Uncuffed endotracheal tubes depend on the physiologic cuff created by the natural shape of the child's trachea.[1] During volume controlled ventilation, if excessive air escapes around the endotracheal tube, the clinician cannot be certain that the tidal volume desired is being delivered to the child's lung and thus the patient may not be adequately ventilated. Measures of tidal volume derived from the ventilator may be inaccurate because the lost volume escaping outside the ventilation circuit is unaccounted for.[8] This potential for air leak also presents a challenge to measuring expired end-tidal carbon dioxide accurately because the children do not exhale completely via the circuit. However, advances in cuffed endotracheal tubes designed specifically for the pediatric airway have proved effective and safe for use in infants and small children.[8] Pediatric clinicians should be aware of and monitor airway leaks at all times because the efficacy of ventilation can be significantly affected by seemingly benign maneuvers. Assessment of ventilation should be done after routine care that may alter the amount of volume escaping around the endotracheal tube and circuit; for example, alterations to the endotracheal tube or repositioning of the child in bed.

Target tidal volumes of 6 mL/kg are recommended for lung protective ventilation.[9] The Acute Respiratory Distress Syndrome Network (ARDSnet) trial showed that limiting the tidal volume to 6 mL/kg in adults with acute respiratory distress syndrome led to a 22% reduction in mortality. In contrast with using a predicted weight calculation of tidal volume in the ARDSnet trail, tidal volume settings are titrated to actual weight in children. Using actual weight to target a tidal volume of 6 mL/kg in children when there is failure to thrive or obesity may alter the tidal volume exposure to the lung.

Ventilators are able to display measures of the tidal volumes delivered to the lung during inspiration and the volume returned in patient expiration. These measurements can be obtained either from flow sensors placed at the end of the patient's endotracheal tube or from flow sensors located at the inlet and outlet of the ventilator. When tidal volume is measured at the level of the ventilator the accuracy of these tidal volume measures may not reflect volume delivery to the lung. In children, the smaller tidal volumes delivered can be affected by ventilator circuit compliance. Compliant ventilator circuits can dampen a large portion of the tidal volume delivered, making it difficult for the clinician to know accurately how much of the breath was received by the patient. Some ventilator technology compensates for this anticipated volume loss in the circuit by using mathematical calculations to estimate and correct the values displayed. However, studies comparing ventilator-derived measurements with actual measurements taken at the level of the patient airway have suggest that tidal volume delivery can be overestimated as much as 56%.[10] The addition of devices to the ventilator circuit, such as closed suction catheter systems and connections for end-tidal carbon dioxide monitoring, may affect the accuracy of these measurements by further altering the compliance of the circuit and adding dead space volume.[10]

The importance of volume-targeted ventilation parameters and the challenges of accurate measures of volume in children demand that critical care nurses understand and interpret technological parameters and feedback and also the clinical tolerance derived from thorough clinical assessment. Close hourly assessment of breath sounds, presence of endotracheal tube leaks, endotracheal tube positioning, chest movement, responses to care activities, and work of breathing are essential in ensuring safe and effective mechanical ventilation for children.

NONINVASIVE VENTILATION CONSIDERATIONS

The trend toward noninvasive ventilation in adults is growing and the use of noninvasive ventilation in pediatric care has increased in parallel.[11] However, the indications, application, and complications associated with noninvasive ventilation for children can be different from the adult experience. There is a paucity of literature to guide best practices for noninvasive ventilation in children and again there is reliance on evidence developed from the adult experience.[12,13]

The technology and devices available for noninvasive ventilation therapy have been largely designed for adults and often require adaptation for children. Adults have multiple interfaces available to them: masks (full face, nasal, partial, total), prongs, pillows, oral appliances, and tents, to name a few. There are significantly fewer options available for children. It has been shown that the success of noninvasive ventilation is directly influenced by the success of the interface used.[14,15] Ventilator manufacturers are also beginning to modify software to better meet the needs of children. Interfaces can be modified to suit a dual-limb system, alternatively software can be modified to accommodate the lower flow rates needed to allow ventilators to be synchronous with the pediatric patient in a noninvasive mode. This area of ventilation is still evolving in children.

Some of the adult interface options are not recommended for children. For example, young or weak children are unlikely to remove a full-face mask when feeling nauseous, thus increasing their risk for aspiration.[15,16] Nasal masks reduce this risk and also provide opportunities for positive oral stimulation in children; for example, a soother and non-nutritive sucking in infants. However, children are not small adults and as such it can be difficult to provide the required device adaptations for age-related variations in anatomy, respiratory physiology, and specific childhood disorders.

To date, there are limited options for pediatric sizes of nasal masks available in Canada for children 3 kg to 25 kg. This limitation has led to the need for some unconventional, creative, and individually derived solutions. Device fit, skin integrity, leaks, and comfort are challenges in pediatric noninvasive ventilation. Poorly fitting masks can lead to pressure sores, leaking of air into eyes causing discomfort and potential corneal injury, and delayed adaptation and refusal to wear the mask.

Developmental factors can also influence noninvasive ventilation success. Children may resist closing their mouths and struggle with the sensation of positive airways pressure. Noninvasive devices are designed to compensate for leaks around the mask by increasing the flow delivered to the patient, thus maintaining the prescribed pressure.[17] This additional flow can be problematic in children. It diminishes sensitivity of the device, can negatively affect the child's synchronicity with the device, and ultimately decreases the efficacy of treatment. Frequent assessments of tolerance to the therapy, interval checking of the skin integrity under the device, application of a pressure/friction-reducing dressing to reddened areas on the skin, meticulous oral hygiene with non–alcohol-based products, application of artificial tears or lubricating eye ointment for eye protection, and thorough pain and sedation assessments with validated measures are important nursing interventions for noninvasively ventilated children. Many children are on spontaneous-breathing modes, so sedation and analgesia for comfort should be titrated to ensure that the child's respiratory drive is not compromised.

Frequent reevaluation of therapy and the interface device is needed both in the intermediate (fluid shifts that influence mask fit, decreased skin perfusion associated with critical illness that may increase risks for skin breakdown) and in the longer term (growth of child) in order to maximize adaptation to the therapy and ensure that support for growth and development is optimized. This reevaluation is very different from that in the adult population, in which a sleep study may provide information for a therapy that may not be reevaluated for many months or years. Considerations for long-term ventilation support of children are discussed later.

CONSIDERATION FOR LONG-TERM VENTILATION IN CHILDREN

The numbers of children being discharged home receiving long-term ventilation continues to increase exponentially.[18] This increase has been catalyzed by improvements in acute illness management and advances in medical technology that have resulted in the survival of children with previously life-threatening or terminal conditions. These same advances have made it possible to facilitate the transition of these children to the community despite their medical complexity. This transition has allowed children and families to realize the benefits of care at home and has enhanced the integration of these technologically dependent children into the community. This transition has also resulted in changes to the population of children seeking acute illness care in critical care units. Although these children and families start their ventilation journey in a critical care environment their ongoing care is provided mainly in the community. There are unique challenges in the care of ventilated children and their families as they transition from acute illness to chronic ventilator-dependent status.

Children requiring long-term mechanical ventilation comprise a heterogeneous population in terms of disease, prognosis, and family resources, which makes determining the ideal ventilation modality an individualized process tailored to the needs of individual children and the clinical context. Knowledge of the clinical diagnosis, prognosis, and psychosocial impact on family life and available resources in the home all influence the determination of the ventilation plan of care as well as the holistic care of the child. The 5 main modes used for long-term mechanical ventilation are (1) positive pressure ventilation via a tracheostomy, (2) noninvasive positive pressure ventilation with a mask, (3) diaphragmatic pacing, (4) negative pressure ventilation, and (5) mouthpiece ventilation. The particular device within each of these 5 categories used in any specific case is usually subject to the patient's individual requirements, as well as the local center's experience and resource availability.[3]

Long-term ventilation support for children can be offered via invasive or noninvasive methods. Noninvasive long-term ventilation support is associated with fewer home care complications and is the therapy of choice when transitioning a child to long-term care who is intubated and ventilated to extubated and ventilated.[19] Many of these children and families transition to home from the critical care unit or from the acute-inpatient area depending on the predictability of their individualized needs and complexity of the medical interventions involved. Regardless of their location within the health care organization, these children and their families require the support of critical care nurses in the delivery and titration of plans of care.

If a child cannot separate from ventilation or is unable to wean from noninvasive support during waking hours, then a tracheostomy is considered. Tracheostomy requires the child to undergo a surgical procedure and the family to learn the care and management of both the tracheostomy and the ventilation technology. This process requires that significant resources be established in the home, including the addition of trained health care providers and 24-h/d monitoring and surveillance of the child. The addition of oxygen, suction equipment, and any related supportive therapies (feeding pumps, nebulized medication treatments) add to the burden of learning and the impact of health care technology in the home.

Critical care nurses may be less familiar with or have limited experience with the portable home care equipment. This lack of familiarity necessitates a close collaboration with home ventilation services to ensure that critical care providers are competent not only to manage the child's transition to the home care technology but also to support the family caregiver learning and consolidation of the skills needed to care for the child after discharge. Invasively ventilated patients require an extensive list of equipment when transitioning home. Home equipment is often introduced at a critical care bedside to test and ensure suitability for care after discharge. For young and/or weak patients, home units may pose issues if the child is not able to trigger the device. This situation requires modification to settings and possibly waiting for child to become stronger, thus delaying discharge. Once a child is safely transitioned to a portable unit, a 1-week to 2-week period of stability is recommended before discharge can proceed.[3,19]

Home care practices can differ from acute care techniques. This difference can lead to confusion for family learning and among the health care team. Careful and thorough communication, documentation, and evaluation of the child's plan of care, the learning plan for family and community providers, competency-based evaluation of skills, core multidisciplinary teams, and interval review of goals are important nursing interventions to ensure skill development for the family and to establish sustainable care routines that are easily transferred to the home environment.

The preparation required for invasive and for noninvasive ventilation in the community differ. Noninvasive preparation is simpler because the learning associated with caring for a tracheostomy is not required. Nevertheless, individual children and families may have unique learning needs, and timelines for discharge preparation can vary significantly. Children requiring noninvasive ventilation are often transitioned out of the critical care setting once stable and their preparation continues in a less intense ward or rehabilitation environment. These children can sometimes be transitioned in stages to a step-down unit or a ward where the atmosphere and pace of care is designed for parental participation and hands-on learning.

Children who remain in the critical care unit can potentially to be exposed to continued stressors of day and night sleep disruptions, multiple providers, and lack of privacy, which can prolong recovery and adaptation for children and families. Critical care nurses must intentionally evaluate and modify the care environment and routine care processes in order to minimize the disruption of routine critical care activities and maximize flexibility for family learning and caregiving. The support of social workers, spiritual and community resources, transitional care specialists, and advanced practice nurse coordinators can support modifications that support transition for these children.

In addition, there are significant social, financial, and emotional burdens associated with caring for a complex technologically dependent child at home.[20] Support for the child's ongoing development by engaging community programs, rehabilitative services, and social assistance programs should be established before discharge and evaluated frequently as the child grows. Having a strong relationship between the family, the primary community medical team, and the critical care/home ventilation team is important because children on home ventilation have an increased likelihood of returning to critical care for episodes of acute illness.[21] Early and ongoing discussions with the family about expectations and goals of care are important to ensure informed decision making in the event of a crisis. Some evidence exists to suggest that health care professionals may underestimate the quality of life of ventilator-dependent children and end-of-life directives may be unduly influenced by the personal beliefs of health care professionals.[22] Open and ongoing dialogue with the child and family's primary provider team and consideration of the involvement of a palliative expert is advisable as a proactive approach to planning for both unanticipated and predictable challenges in the long term for these fragile children.[23]

DEVELOPMENTAL CONSIDERATIONS FOR VENTILATED CHILDREN

Across all developmental stages of childhood, critical illness and medical fragility are frightening and highly stressful for children. It is important to acknowledge the impact this stress can have on developing children and dedicate resources and focus to mitigating the psychosocial impacts of ventilation. The limitations present in a critical care environment and the diversity of the individual needs of each ventilated child necessitate creative solutions for supporting the children's developmental needs. There is evidence linking prolonged hospitalization with increased incidence of developmental delays.[24] The environmental limitations identified include sensory overload, sleep deprivation, separation from family, multiple caregivers, and lack of access to normal developmental experiences.[25,26] Areas where health care providers can make a positive impact for children include designing care to maximize child participation both in care activities and in decision making appropriate to the child's developmental and cognitive abilities, information sharing paced by the child's needs, and active support for the achievement of developmental skills and milestones.

Exposure to the medical world of a critical care unit is confusing and frightening. Children experience the environment differently at different stages of development (**Table 1**). In a high-stimulus, high-acuity, and high-volume space where there are numerous health care providers interacting in the children's care, children are dealing with the direct impact of their own medical needs and also managing a great many psychological stressors. Studies reveal that the number of invasive procedures experienced by a child is positively associated with the level of stress, anxiety, and fear experienced during and following hospitalization.[27–29] In particular, some studies have found that the number of invasive procedures is predictive of the child's psychological distress, manifested in symptoms of depression, anxiety, fear, and posttraumatic stress.[22,27,29] Ventilation and the associated care of endotracheal tubes, suctioning, ventilator alarms, and disruptions are among the chief sources of invasive stressful experiences for critically ill children.

It is important that ventilated children are supported to become active participants in their care. Simple modifications nurses can make to routine care, such as not performing painful procedures on sleeping children, build trust and engage the children more fully in their experiences.[32] Children, including young infants, can be provided with explanations and anticipatory cues and guidance to help build trust and understanding, and to facilitate the mobilization of coping skills. Sharing accurate information at the child's developmental level can help develop trusting relationships with the health care team and alleviate fear.[33] For toddlers and older children, repeating explanations and addressing concerns helps to build cumulative understanding and anticipation matched to the expectations of the procedure or activity. Regardless of the medical procedure, the key elements of effective preparation are (1) the provision of developmentally appropriate information, (2) the encouragement of emotional expression, and (3) the formation of a trusting relationship with a health care professional.[34–36] These explanations should include sensations that the child can expect to experience, including sights, sounds, smells, and feelings, and the clarification of fears or misconceptions.[37–39] For ventilation cares, preparation for the sensation of

Table 1
Developmental considerations for ventilated children

Consideration	Infants (0–18 mo)	Toddlers (18–36 mo)	Preschool (3–6 y)	School Age (6–13 y)	Adolescents (13–18 y)
Developmental theories	Trust vs mistrust[45] Sensorimotor[46]	Autonomy vs shame and doubt[45] Sensorimotor/preoperational[46]	Initiative vs guilt[45] Preoperational thinking[46]	Industry vs inferiority[45] Concrete operations[46]	Identity vs role confusion[45] Formal operations[46]
Frame of mind	• Is the world good? • Can I trust? • Explores the world through moving, touching, and tasting	• "I want to do it" "Mine" • Asserting independence, but still dependent • Not logical thinkers • Primary task is asking "Am I good or bad?"	• Building confidence in self and figuring out own abilities • Magical thinking dominates. "If I am good they won't give me a needle"	• Independence growing • School very important • Able to help with care • Logical thinkers • Can understand the body and reasons for medical care/equipment in simple terms	• Peers, friends, social, and intimate relationships very important • Creating own identity • Able to think about abstract ideas and the future • Increased body concerns
Hospital stressors and fears	• Limited opportunities for positive touch, consistent care and attention • Risk of decreased trust with the world caused by limited or adverse hospital experiences • Caregivers worried about germs so exploration is sometimes limited	• Separation from parents • Fear of abandonment • Stranger anxiety • Loss of independence • Change in routine • Unfamiliar environment • Immobility • Risk of self-doubt	• Hospitalization as a form of punishment • Fear of separation from parents • Fear of abandonment • Fantasy and magical thinking • Fear of body mutilation • Immobility • Misconceptions about medical experiences	• Disruption of normal routine • Fear of body mutilation; loss of body function • Hospitalization as a form of punishment • Loss of competence or control • Fears pain • Fears death • Fears anesthesia	• Loss of independence • Lack of privacy • Decreased social interactions • Loss of control • Body mutilation and body image • Fear of social rejection and/or lack of peer acceptance • Future capabilities • Developing trusting relationships • Fear of death

Possible interventions	<ul><li>Maximize parental involvement</li><li>Provide positive touch and attention</li><li>Provide play opportunities</li><li>Allow to explore through moving, touching, and tasting (if appropriate)</li><li>Provide opportunities to sit, stand, walk (when appropriate)</li><li>Provide different nonmedical stimuli; eg, mobile, music, rattles, time out of the PICU</li></ul>	<ul><li>Maximize parental involvement</li><li>Facilitate medical play</li><li>Provide accurate preparatory information</li><li>Teach planned coping strategies</li><li>Provide play opportunities</li><li>Provide distraction</li><li>Provide positive touch and attention</li><li>Provide different nonmedical stimuli; eg, iPad, music, toys, crafts, time out of the PICU</li><li>Provide simple options to ensure child is able to make choices</li></ul>	<ul><li>Maximize parental involvement</li><li>Provide opportunities for medical play</li><li>Provide accurate and simple preparatory information</li><li>Teach planned coping strategies; eg, blowing bubbles, singing songs</li><li>Provide play opportunities; eg, crafts, games, toys, iPad</li><li>Provide distraction</li><li>Help children make choices</li><li>Ensure communication aids are offered</li></ul>	<ul><li>Maximize parental involvement</li><li>Ensure children are prepared for and involved in procedures</li><li>Provide opportunities for medical play</li><li>Involve child in understanding body and medical needs</li><li>Teach coping strategies; eg, deep breathing, guided imagery</li><li>Encourage choices; eg, mask vs IV</li><li>Provide age-appropriate activities; eg, TV, crafts, toys, games, puzzles, iPad</li><li>Help children with ways to share their medical needs with peers</li><li>Ensure communication aids are offered</li></ul>	<ul><li>Communicate honestly</li><li>Provide privacy</li><li>Respect independence</li><li>Ensure they are involved in care and given opportunities to make choices</li><li>Address body image, sexual image, and future concerns</li><li>Provide medical preparation</li><li>Provide opportunities for follow-up discussion and guidance</li><li>Provide age-appropriate activities; eg, video games, iPad, crafts, TV, music</li><li>Ensure communication aids are offered</li></ul>

Abbreviations: IV, intravenous; PICU, paediatric intensive care unit.
Data from Refs.[29–31]

suction, elicitation of cough, and pressure are therefore important. For example, a 7-year-old needing noninvasive ventilation might be fearful of the mask, thinking that it might make it hard to breathe.

For infants and children attached to ventilators, experiences that support motor skill development can be limited.[40] Exposure to diverse environments for learning are confined to the care space; children are not handled or held in arms as they would if healthy and they may be restrained at times in order to maintain the safety of necessary invasive medical devices. Critical care nurses can help support development for ventilated children in several ways, such as providing appropriate toys to watch passively and interact with actively when able. There can be many opportunities for play in critical care because play incorporates any activity that the child spontaneously engages in and finds enjoyable.[41,42] Play helps to normalize the hospital environment, has been shown to decrease anxiety, and can provide opportunity for individual expression.[43,44]

Support of communication and language skills development are particularly challenging for ventilated children. Alternative modes of communication for intubated and ventilated children include sign language, which can be learned as young as 8 months of age; the use of a tablet, communication board, or pen and paper; and patterned eye movements for children experiencing paralysis. All these possibilities are feasible with cognitively aware children, but they do require practice, patience, and creativity on both the child's and nurse's parts. Children with long-term ventilation via tracheostomy many need a combination of the methods of communication listed earlier, depending on their age, cognitive development, and neurologic status.[43] The use of a speaking valve, when medically appropriate, has helped many children to vocalize. Focus on helping children communicate is essential because it gives children an opportunity to guide their care and gain an element of control that is desperately needed in their dependent state.[32]

When possible, ventilated children benefit from a core group of primary nurses being assigned to work with them. Working with the same child enables nurses to learn the child's behavioral cues, responses to interventions, and ability to cope. This approach helps children feel more stable and allows each day to be more predictable, enhancing their trust.[32] This constancy is enhanced by an informative and detailed care plan that includes information on the child's likes and dislikes, how the child acts when they are overstressed or tired, and how the parents want to be engaged in their child's care.[32]

Children must continue to learn, grow, and play during critical illness and should not be overly hampered by the necessity of ventilation support providing their medical condition allows and their individual cognitive, social, and physical levels of functioning are respected. A plan of care that incorporates the specific developmental needs of the child's stage and cognitive level, creative approaches to care delivery, and the engagement of the family's knowledge of the child, as well as the expertise of the interdisciplinary team, can help to support ventilated children to maintain their developmental trajectories.

SUMMARY

Support of oxygenation and ventilation is an integral component of expert critical care nursing for children. Understanding the unique experience of children and the particular assessments, challenges, and strategies for managing maturing physiology, and recognizing the issues related to childhood pulmonary care, ensures the well-being of the children and supports the adaptation for families. The success of ventilation therapy in children is greatly influenced by the collaboration between the health care team, the children, and the parents. Parents can inform and lead in identifying strategies for soothing and supporting the children's adaptation to therapy, whereas the health care team brings experience in symptom management and anticipatory knowledge about the trajectory of care and risk mitigation. Together, the child and family, the critical care team, partners, and multidisciplinary experts must acknowledge the unique challenges of ventilation interventions for children and work to remove risk and support recovery of these vulnerable patients.

REFERENCES

1. Curley MQ, Grant JC. Pulmonary critical care problems. In: Curley MQ, Maloney-Harmon P, editors. Critical care nursing of infants and children. 2nd edition. Philadelphia: WB Saunders; 2001. p. 655–94.
2. Kendirli T, Kavaz A, Yalaki Z, et al. Mechanical ventilation in children. Turk J Pediatr 2006;48(4):32–3.
3. Paulides F, Plötz F, Verweij-van den Oudenrijn L, et al. Thirty years of home mechanical ventilation in children: escalating need for pediatric intensive care beds. Intensive Care Med 2012;38:847–52.
4. Slutsky AS. Ventilator-induced lung injury: from barotrauma to biotrauma. Respir Care 2005;50:646–59.
5. Duyndam A, Ista E, Houmes JR, et al. Invasive ventilation modes in children: a systematic review and meta-analysis. Crit Care 2011;15:R24.
6. Cheifetz I. Invasive and noninvasive pediatric mechanical. Respir Care 2003; 48(4):442–53.
7. Randolph AG. Management of acute lung injury and acute respiratory distress syndrome in children. Crit Care Med 2009;37:2448–54.
8. Taylor C. Pediatric cuffed endotracheal tubes: an evolution of care. Ochsner J 2011;11:52–6.
9. The Acute Respiratory Distress Syndrome Network. Ventilation with lower tidal volumes as compared with traditional tidal volumes for acute lung injury and the acute respiratory distress syndrome. N Engl J Med 2000;342:1301–8.
10. Cheifetz I, Cannon M, Cornell J, et al. Tidal volume measurements for ventilated infants should be measured with a pneumotachometer placed at the endotracheal tube. Am J Respir Crit Care Med 2000;162:2109–12.
11. Demaret P, Mulder A, Loeck I, et al. Non-invasive ventilation is useful in paediatric intensive care units if children are appropriately selected and carefully monitored. Acta Paediatr 2015;104(9):861–87.
12. Abadesso C, Nunes P, Silvestre C, et al. Non-invasive ventilation in acute respiratory failure in children. Pediatr Rep 2012;4(2):e16.
13. Chatwin M, Tan H, Bush A, et al. Long term non-invasive ventilation in children: impact on survival and transition to adult care. PLoS One 2015;10(5):e0125839.
14. Carroll A, Olmstead D, Klein J, et al. Mask issues in pediatric non-invasive positive pressure ventilation: a Focus Group. Am J Respir Crit Care Med 2015;191: A5060.
15. Mayordomo-Colunga J, Medina A, Rey R, et al. Predictive factors of non invasive ventilation failure in critically ill children: a prospective epidemiological study. Intensive Care Med 2009;35(3):527–36.
16. Norregaard O. Noninvasive ventilation in children. Eur Respir J 2002;20(5): 1332–42.

17. Nava S, Ambrosino N, Bruschi C, et al. Physiological effects of flow and pressure triggering during non-invasive mechanical ventilation in patients with chronic obstructive pulmonary disease. Thorax 1997;52:249–54.

18. Dhilln JS, Frewen TC, Singh NC, et al. Chronic mechanical ventilation-dependent children in Canada. Paediatr Child Health 1996;1(2):111–6.

19. Wallis C, Paton JY, Beaton S, et al. Children on long-term ventilatory support: 10 years of progress. Arch Dis Child 2011;96:998–1002.

20. Carnevale FA, Alexander E, Davis M, et al. Daily living with distress and enrichment: the moral experience of families with ventilator-assisted children at home. Pediatrics 2006;117(1):e48–60.

21. Graham RJ, Fleegler EW, Robinson WM. Chronic ventilator need in the community: a 2005 pediatric census of Massachusetts. Pediatrics 2007;119(6):e1280–7.

22. Gowans M, Keenan HT, Bratton SL. The population prevalence of children receiving invasive home ventilation in Utah. Pediatr Pulmonol 2007;42(3):231–6.

23. Rapoport A, Beune L, Weingarten K, et al. Living life to the fullest: early integration of palliative care into the lives of children with chronic complex conditions. Curr Pediatr Rev 2012;8(2):152–65.

24. Lehner D, Sadler L. Toddler developmental delays after extensive hospitalization: primary care practitioner guidelines. Pediatr Nurs 2015;41(5):236–42.

25. Kudchadkar S, Othman A, Punjabi N. Sleep of critically ill children in the pediatric intensive care unit: a systematic review. Sleep Med Rev 2014;18:103–10.

26. Forsner M, Jansson L, Sørlie V. The experience of being ill as narrated by hospitalized children aged 7-10 years with short-term illness. J Child Health Care 2005; 9(2):153–65.

27. Rennick JE, Johnston CC, Dougherty G, et al. Children's psychological responses after critical illness and exposure to invasive technology. J Dev Behav Pediatr 2002;23(3):133–44.

28. Rennick JE, Morin I, Kim D, et al. Identifying children at high risk for psychological sequelae after pediatric intensive care unit hospitalization. Pediatr Crit Care Med 2004;5(4):358–63.

29. Salmela M, Salantera S, Aronen E. Child reported hospital fears in 4 to 6 year old children. Pediatr Nurs 2009;35(5):269–303.

30. Coyne I. Children's experiences of hospitalization. J Child Health Care 2006; 10(4):326–36.

31. Rollins JA, Bolig R, Mahan CC. Meeting children's psychosocial needs across the health-care continuum. Austin (TX): Pro-Ed; 2005.

32. Warner J, Norwood S. Psychosocial concerns of the ventilator-dependent child in the pediatric intensive care unit. AACN Clin Issues Crit Care Nurs 1991;2(3): 432–45.

33. Stevenson MD, Bivins CM, O'Brien K, et al. Child Life intervention during angiocatheter insertion in the pediatric emergency department. Pediatr Emerg Care 2005;21(11):712–8.

34. Tideman ME, Clatworthy S. Anxiety responses of 5- to 11-year-old children during and after hospitalization. J Pediatr Nurs 1990;5(5):334–43.

35. O'Connor-Von S. Preparing children for surgery: an integrative research review. AORN J 2000;71(2):334–43.

36. Campbell LA, Kirkpatrick SE, Berry CC, et al. Preparing children with congenital heart disease for cardiac surgery. J Pediatr Psychol 1995;20(3):313–28.

37. Lynch M. Preparing children for day surgery. Child Health Care 1994;23(2): 75–85.

38. Brewer S, Gleditsch SL, Syblik D, et al. Pediatric anxiety: child life intervention in day surgery. J Pediatr Nurs 2006;21(1):13–22.

39. Kratz A. Preoperative education: preparing patients for a positive experience. J Post Anesth Nurs 1993;8(4):270–5.

40. Glader LJ, Palfrey JS. Care of the child assisted by technology. Pediatr Rev 2009; 30:439–45.

41. Fisher EP. The impact of play on development: a meta-analysis. Play Culture 1992;5(2):159–81.

42. Jiang D, Morrison GJ. The influence of long-term tracheostomy on speech and language development in children. Int J Pediatr Otorhinolaryngol 2003;67:S21.

43. Norris AE, Aroian KJ, Warren S, et al. Interactive performance and focus groups with adolescents: the power of play. Res Nurs Health 2012;35:671–9.

44. Li WH, Chung JO, Ho KY, et al. Play interventions to reduce anxiety and negative emotions in hospitalized children. BMC Pediatr 2016;16:36.

45. Erikson EH. Childhood and society. London (United Kingdom): WW Norton & Company; 1993.

46. Piaget J. The construction of reality in the child (Vol. 82). Oxford (United Kingdom): Routledge; 2013.

Special Considerations in Neonatal Mechanical Ventilation

Stacey Dalgleish, MN, NP[a], Linda Kostecky, RN, BN[a],
Irina Charania, RRT[b],*

KEYWORDS

- Neonatal • Mechanical ventilation • Interprofessional • Teamwork
- Patient-centered care

KEY POINTS

- Front-line nursing staff have a key role in skilled management of mechanically ventilated neonates.
- Communication of assessments and observations regarding changes in patient status allow timely and appropriate care decisions to be made by the interprofessional team.
- Interprofessional teamwork is key to ensuring optimal management of ventilated neonates.
- Successful management of ventilated neonates requires a comprehensive approach to care, with a focus on the patient as a whole, rather than on a single organ system.
- Parental involvement in the neonatal intensive care unit is extremely important to patient outcomes, and front-line nurses provide critical supports to parents during each infant's stay in the neonatal intensive care unit.

INTRODUCTION

Over the past decades many advances have been made in how care is provided to neonatal intensive care unit (NICU) patients. Neonatal nurses are among the most constant and consistent care providers that neonates encounter during the NICU stay and respiratory support remains a mainstay of neonatal intensive care. Mechanical ventilation has proved to be essential to the survival of most extremely premature neonates and will continue to play a key role in neonatal intensive care.[1] Although lifesaving, neonatal ventilation is associated with acute and chronic lung and airway complications, including but not limited to air leaks, atelectasis, infection, and bronchopulmonary dysplasia.[1–3]

---

[a] Neonatal Intensive Care Unit, Foothills Medical Centre, 1403 29 Street Northwest, Calgary, Alberta, Canada; [b] Advanced Technical Skills Simulation Laboratory, University of Calgary, 3330 Hospital Drive Northwest, Calgary, Alberta T2N 1N4, Canada
* Corresponding author.
E-mail address: irina.charania2@ucalgary.ca

Crit Care Nurs Clin N Am 28 (2016) 477–498
http://dx.doi.org/10.1016/j.cnc.2016.07.007
0899-5885/16/© 2016 Elsevier Inc. All rights reserved.

ccnursing.theclinics.com

Antenatal steroids, surfactant treatment, and new strategies for neonatal respiratory care have dramatically changed the presentation, clinical course, and long-term outcomes for neonates with respiratory illness.[4] Focus has expanded from ensuring survival to reducing the incidence of chronic lung disease and neurodevelopmental impairment.[5] Unlike other organs, the neonatal lung completes a significant portion of its development at the end of gestation and postnatally.[6,7] The neonatal lung has the ability to repair but is also highly susceptible to lung injury. Neonates present with different pathophysiology compared with pediatric and adult populations. In addition, infants of different gestations may require different ventilation strategies based on their individual disease state.

Nursing care of ventilated infants shares many features with the care of any other age group of ventilated patients. The overarching goal of neonatal mechanical ventilation is to support adequate gas exchange with minimal adverse effects on the infant's lungs, hemodynamics, and brain.[5,8] The unique characteristics of infants pose additional challenges and opportunities for affecting health outcomes. In particular, the infant's state of rapid growth and development and the exquisitely close interdependence between their respiratory systems and all other body functions require a high level of assessment expertise to discern how to interpret subtle changes in an infant's condition. It is not a set of lungs that clinicians are treating, it is a critically ill infant, who is part of a family, and who requires mechanical ventilation for support. Expert nursing care of this fragile population requires close collaboration with medical staff, respiratory therapists, dieticians, and other members of the interprofessional team, and (perhaps most importantly) should include the infant's parents.[9–14]

Every infant receiving mechanical ventilation in a NICU receives care from a team dedicated to ensuring that the best possible outcome is achieved given the resources that are currently available. Survival and neurodevelopmental outcomes of premature babies depend on a multitude of variables. This article focuses on current best practices for the care of critically ill infants receiving mechanical ventilation.

COMMUNICATION

Effective communication and teamwork among the care providers cannot be overlooked. In the pursuit of optimal health outcomes team members must go beyond cooperation. They must collaborate by coordinating their efforts and resources in order to achieve a mutually desired goal.

The essential characteristics of high-performing teams have been documented extensively in the patient safety literature, with effective teamwork being identified as a key determinant of quality care and patient safety.[15–17] The ability of a team to establish and maintain a shared mental model is vital for ensuring that resources are effectively coordinated. Leonard and Frankel[15] described the basic elements of teamwork and communication. These elements include effective organizational and clinical leadership behaviors, structured communication strategies, effective critical language, situational awareness, and perhaps most importantly psychological safety. Miller and colleagues[16] identified that effective health care team performance is highly dependent on nurses and their ability to successfully transfer critical information. Nurse-to-nurse communication and hand-off reports provide vital information for the oncoming caregiver to be aware of what is usual for each individual infant, which facilitates early and appropriate responses to subtle and/or rapid changes in the infants' clinical status.

For health care providers caring for mechanically ventilated patients, a significant communication challenge is navigating the vast and often industry-driven, proprietary terminology that must be understood in order to provide optimal therapies.[18] For the purposes of this article, common language is proposed to facilitate understanding and allow smoother interprofessional collaboration. Understanding of neonatal lung disease and management strategies is continuously evolving[19] and it is paramount that all team members practice according to current evidence. This article describes underpinning lung physiology and mechanical ventilation strategies, and identifies unique nursing strategies to support ventilated neonates.

OVERVIEW OF FETAL AND NEONATAL LUNG DEVELOPMENT

A common understanding of fetal and neonatal lung anatomy and physiology is a necessary foundation facilitating effective communication about mechanical ventilation among NICU health care providers. The following overview provides a brief context of underlying principles in fetal and neonatal lung development (**Fig. 1**) before discussing strategies for care of mechanically ventilated neonates.

Fetal lung development occurs in 5 stages with imprecise boundaries, beginning with the embryonic stage, which encompasses the first 6 weeks of gestation. This stage includes the appearance of the lung bud and main pulmonary arteries. Gestational weeks 6 to 16 are referred to as the pseudoglandular stage. During this stage all the conducting airways leading to the gas exchange zones of the lung are formed, including the associated vasculature. The canalicular stage occurs between weeks 16 and 24. It is characterized by significant capillary multiplication and network formation. This newly formed capillary network begins to approach the primitive air spaces by 23 weeks, creating an early gas exchange membrane. The canalicular stage is

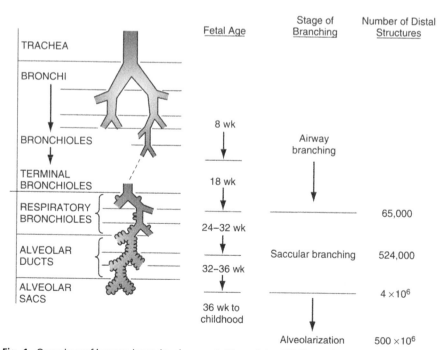

Fig. 1. Overview of human lung development. (*From* Jobe AH, Kamath-Rayne BD. Fetal lung development and surfactant. In: Creasy RK, Resnik R, Iams JD, et al, editors. Creasy and Resnik's maternal-fetal medicine: principles and practice. Elsevier Health Sciences; 2014. p. 177.)

followed by the saccular stage, which starts around 24 weeks and ends around 40 weeks. During this stage, type II alveolar cells begin producing surfactant at around 26 weeks, and surfactant excretion typically begins around 30 weeks. True alveoli begin to form around 32 weeks and are uniformly present by 38 weeks. The last stage of lung development occurs primarily after birth; it is called the alveolarization stage. Human lung development continues until about 8 years of age, with 85% of alveoli forming between birth and 2 years of age.

Note that, beginning in the canalicular phase, lung formation and growth begin to be significantly affected by mechanical forces in the form of transpulmonary pressure resulting from fetal lung fluid that is excreted by pulmonary epithelial cells, cyclical stretching forces created by fetal breathing movements, and in pathologic states by other sources of intrathoracic or extrathoracic pressure.[20–24] It has been hypothesized that lung hypoplasia is directly linked to a reduction in lung expansion from a loss of lung fluid volume.[25] In addition, in-utero fetal lung development occurs in a fairly hypoxic environment.[22,23] These points are important to keep in mind in the following discussions about managing ventilation and oxygenation for neonatal patients. The disruption of fetal lung development through premature birth has been shown to result in adverse pulmonary outcomes that last throughout the lifetime.[26] Even disruptions that are a result of late prematurity have been linked to increased morbidity in survivors.[22]

At birth the lung must quickly transition from a fluid-filled organ with no meaningful role in gas exchange to an air-filled organ that is solely responsible for the gas exchange required to sustain life.[27] One of the key markers of effective transition and lung function after birth in healthy neonates is the establishment of functional residual capacity (FRC).[27] In a healthy term newborn, an FRC of approximately 30 mL/kg of body weight is established within 2 to 6 hours after birth, depending on the mode of delivery.[28] FRC is essential for normal lung function because it optimizes gas exchange surface area by stabilizing the alveoli, and this is a primary factor in ensuring optimal oxygenation and removal of carbon dioxide (CO_2). Optimal FRC is achieved when the alveoli are neither underdistended nor overdistended.

Underinflation may produce or prolong the existence of both shunts and dead space in the lungs. Shunting is characterized by adequate perfusion with inadequate ventilation. Dead spaces occur in areas of collapsed alveoli, where inspired air cannot reach the air-gas interface and participate in gas exchange.

In contrast, if alveoli are overdistended, they may contribute to decreased pulmonary blood perfusion through 2 proposed mechanisms. Direct pressure applied to the capillary network could increase resistance and decrease blood flow, or an increase in intrathoracic pressure applied to the heart could decrease cardiac output and pulmonary flow. Therefore, the establishment of an optimal FRC is essential for optimal ventilation and oxygenation to take place.[29] In mechanically ventilated neonates, optimal FRC is controlled by the positive end-expiratory pressure (PEEP) set on the ventilator. Providing mechanical ventilation with a goal of establishing and maintaining optimal FRC using PEEP is commonly referred to as an open lung strategy.[1]

OVERVIEW OF NEONATAL MECHANICAL VENTILATION
Mechanical Ventilation Terminology Overview

A mechanical breath includes an inspiratory and an expiratory phase. The event that prompts the initiation of the inspiratory phase is called a trigger. Inhalation is sustained by either a constant flow (volume-limited ventilation) or a constant pressure (pressure-limited ventilation). The event that prompts the transition to the expiratory phase is called the cycling mechanism. Despite the plethora of proprietary ventilator mode terminology, all mechanical ventilator breaths and modes can be described using these terms.[18,30,31] With the use of common language based on the underlying principles, practitioners are more likely to be successful in achieving a shared mental model and effective communication around mechanical ventilation of the neonate. **Fig. 2** provides a flow chart that bedside practitioners can use to identify and discuss the current mode of ventilation for infants who are able to make spontaneous respiratory efforts.

Historically, neonates have commonly been treated using pressure-limited modes of mechanical ventilation.[5] These modes deliver inhalation to a set pressure, then trigger the exhalation phase. A significant disadvantage of this simple approach is that it is not sensitive to changes in the infant's lung compliance. Pressure-limited ventilation relies on manual adjustment of inflation pressure, with no direct control of tidal volume being possible. Tidal volume is defined as the change in the volume of air in the lungs between when inspiration is initiated and the volume of air in the lungs at the end of the inspiration. Rapid, sometimes dramatic, compliance changes occur following initial inflation, surfactant administration, or resorption of fetal lung fluid. Improved lung compliance, when not quickly identified and responded to with

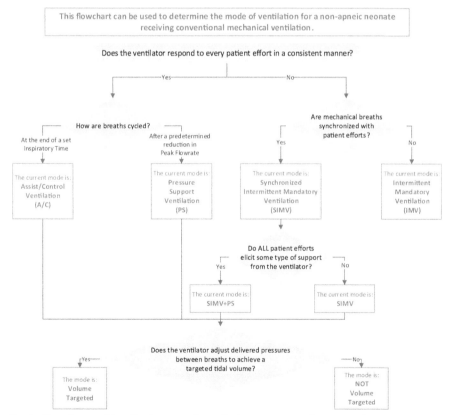

Fig. 2. Flowchart to identify the type of ventilation a non-apneic neonate is receiving. It is a tool to aid communication and the establishment of a shared mental model around mechanical ventilation without reliance on manufacturer terminology.

adjustments in mechanical ventilator settings, commonly results in iatrogenic hyperventilation and lung injury. Lung damage caused by excessive volume delivery is referred to as volutrauma.[2,3,5]

Although both high tidal volumes and high peak pressures are damaging to the neonatal lung,[2,3] high inflation pressures cause lung injury only when they result in excessive tidal volume. Animal research reveals that as few as 6 excessively large breaths could negate the benefits of surfactant therapy.[32] In contrast, insufficient tidal volume may allow the alveoli to remain underinflated. This condition is undesirable because it results in hypercapnia, increased work of breathing, increased oxygen requirement, agitation, fatigue, and/or atelectasis.[5] **Table 1** provides an overview of some of the different types of lung injury applicable to the neonatal lung, and their sources.

Current evidence guides clinicians to first establish FRC, then select a ventilator mode based on the infant's current pathophysiology with a goal to minimize ventilator-induced lung injury.

VENTILATOR MODE SELECTION

Lung protection strategies are based on the concept of distributing tidal volume evenly into an optimally aerated lung.[5,33] Adequate PEEP is described as optimal PEEP. A lung with areas of atelectasis preferentially distributes tidal volume to the aerated portion of the lung. These aerated alveoli are more compliant than atelectatic portions of lung, leading to overdistention and subsequent volutrauma.[1] Uninflated or atelectatic regions experience surfactant deactivation and increased inflammation.[2,3] Uneven forces between inflated and atelectatic regions contribute to further lung damage. Open lung concepts are necessary to prevent lung injury in ventilated neonates while optimizing CO_2 clearance and oxygenation.[34] There exists a balance between providing optimum respiratory support while avoiding overventilation or an unnecessary length of mechanical ventilation time.[35] Bedside assessment and monitoring are key to ensuring that infants are maintained within that balanced, optimal state of respiratory support. Changes in oxygen saturation, oxygen concentration requirements, blood pressure, and level of agitation may indicate that the infant's respiratory support needs are changing; a rapid and effective response is required to bring the baby back into the balanced state, and prevent lung injury.

Another strategy for optimizing mechanical ventilation outcomes in neonates is permissive hypercapnia.[36–39] Permissive hypercapnia is defined as a target $Paco_2$

Table 1	
Types of neonatal lung injury	
Classification of Lung Injury	**Causal Mechanism**
Volutrauma	Overdistension of the lung tissue caused by excessive tidal volume delivery
Atelectrauma	Insufficient end-expiratory pressure leading to excessive shearing forces caused by the repeated collapse and reinflation of lung tissue
Barotrauma	The use of excessive peak inspiratory pressures leading to overdistension and damage of compliant lung tissue
Biotrauma	Damage to lung tissue caused by inflammatory mediators. This inflammatory response can be triggered by either direct injury to lung tissue, often from one or more of the lung injury mechanisms listed in this table, or from an inflammatory response related to an infection

value of greater than 45 mm Hg, with a pH of greater than 7.25. As with other mechanical ventilation strategies, optimal titration is critical to success, and depends on multiple variables, such as perfusion, agitation, kidney function, and other concurrent medical treatments. This rule is especially true in the first 3 days of life, during which $Paco_2$ values of greater than 65 mm Hg have been associated with increased intraventricular hemorrhage risk.[40]

In summary, essential strategies in protecting the neonatal lung during mechanical ventilation include optimizing lung volume, limiting excessive lung expansion, application of appropriate PEEP levels, using shorter inspiratory time and small tidal volumes, and the appropriate use of permissive hypercapnia.[36] Neonatal mechanical ventilators continue to advance; however, better technology alone will not improve outcomes unless used with optimal ventilation strategies and expert supportive care.

NURSING CARE
Intubation

Endotracheal intubation, either elective or emergent, is a potentially lifesaving procedure that can be performed by either the oropharyngeal or nasopharyngeal route.[41,42] There are 5 accepted indications for endotracheal intubation, as outlined in **Box 1**.

All airway management equipment must be ready for an emergent or elective intubation procedure.[41] Essential equipment is outlined in **Box 2**.

The nursing role before and during intubation may include preparation of equipment; provision of comfort to the infant through facilitated tucking[43,44]; positioning for a successful procedure; monitoring of infant tolerance, including vital signs; administration of any preintubation medications; and as parent support. Following the intubation procedure, the nurse continues to monitor and document tolerance of the procedure and the ventilatory mode, note securement of the endotracheal tube, and support the infant emerging from the effects of analgesic/paralytic agents.

Once the intubation decision has been made, the shared goal of the interprofessional team is to prevent and minimize adverse events related to mechanical ventilation, until the infant can be successfully extubated.[45] Simulations may be useful to prepare the interprofessional team to care for the critically ill mechanically ventilated neonate.[46] Potential benefits of practice through simulation in a safe environment include both role rehearsal and ability to identify learning needs.

Unplanned Extubation

An unplanned extubation poses a significant risk of harm to an infant, and should be considered a potentially life-threatening event. Unplanned extubation can cause cardiorespiratory deterioration and other adverse effects, including airway trauma, subglottic stenosis, and ventilator-associated pneumonia (VAP).[47] After the endotracheal tube has been replaced, the infant may experience ventilator-induced lung injury

---

Box 1
Indications for endotracheal intubation

1. Mechanical ventilatory support

2. Airway patency

3. Airway protection

4. Suctioning

5. Surgery

Box 2
Essential equipment for neonatal endotracheal intubation

1. Oxygen source with a blender

2. A self-inflating resuscitation bag or T-piece device

3. Various sizes of face masks

4. Suction device and various sizes of sterile suction catheters

5. Laryngoscope and appropriate blade sizes

6. Endotracheal tubes of sizes 2.0 to 4.0 mm internal diameter

7. Magill forceps (for nasal intubations)

8. Securement device

9. Stethoscope

10. Method to verify endotracheal intubation (CO_2 detection device, end tidal CO_2 monitor)

11. Premedication as ordered

---

in the form of atelectrauma,[2] increased oxygen exposure to bring them back to target oxygenation levels, and prolonged mechanical ventilation days.

Merkel and colleagues[47] report a successful quality improvement intervention to reduce the rate of unplanned extubations in a single NICU. Using staff education and implementing standard practices of care allowed a benchmark of less than 1 unplanned extubation per 100 intubated patient days to be met and sustained. **Box 3** summarizes 4 potentially best practices that can be implemented by interprofessional NICU teams in order to prevent unplanned extubations.

Unplanned extubation should be a safety concern for all NICUs. As with many quality improvement projects, continuous vigilance, staff training, and benchmarking of events are crucial to maintain standards of care.[47]

SUCTIONING

Best practice for endotracheal suctioning is to suction only as needed based on clinical assessment versus performing routine endotracheal suctioning.[48] The indications

---

Box 3
Summary of potentially best practices for the prevention of unplanned extubations in neonates

1. A minimum of 2 experienced caregivers should be involved in procedures such as weighing, patient transfer, and securing endotracheal tubes. One person takes responsibility just for safely maintaining the endotracheal tube, whereas the second person performs required tasks. A very fragile or very active infant may require additional team members (including the parents) to assist so that all handling is done in a safe, controlled manner, with full consideration given to pacing care tasks to the infant's tolerance.

2. Placement of alert cards at the bedside indicating the depth of placement at the gums along with documentation of endotracheal tube position and securement by both the nurse and respiratory therapist during routine care.

3. The use of a commercially available product to optimally secure the endotracheal tube.

4. Every unplanned extubation is reviewed and analyzed for root cause.

for suctioning include visible or audible secretions in the endotracheal tube, coarse or absent respiratory sounds, bradycardia, desaturation, and increased work of breathing. Ventilators with pulmonary mechanics may show a change in tidal volume, minute ventilation, and flow-volume loops when secretions are present.

The lowest possible suction pressure is always recommended for endotracheal suctioning.[41]

- In neonates a maximum of 100 mm Hg pressure is recommended.
- Deep suctioning, defined as passing the suction catheter beyond the end of the endotracheal tube, is not recommended because animal studies have shown a potential for airway damage.[49]
- Gentle, rapid suctioning without instillation of normal saline is indicated.[5]

In one neonatal study, isotonic saline solution instillation resulted in a significantly higher number of bradycardia episodes, desaturations, and increased oxygen requirement with no differences in the characteristics of the secretions.[41]

- Closed suction systems are desirable in that the system is sterile because the infant remains connected to the ventilator at all times without interrupting PEEP, which in turn minimizes changes in oxygen saturation and decreases the degree of atelectasis.[48] In addition, nurses favored the closed system regarding ease of use.[50] Nurses play a pivotal role in supporting neonates during suctioning procedures. Ongoing pain assessment and advocacy for analgesia may be appropriate in individual circumstances. Other nonpharmacologic measures, such as facilitated tucking and developmentally supportive care (eg, oral sucrose, paced care, observation, and response to infant cues) may help to modulate stressful situations for neonates.[51] In a 4-handed endotracheal suctioning strategy,[51] person 1 supports the infant's efforts at self-regulation, such as promoting flexion, allowing finger grasp, or touching the infant gently, while person 2 performs the suctioning procedure. Nurses may guide parents in nonpharmacologic, developmentally supportive techniques that may reduce pain and stress for their infants.

VENTILATOR-ASSOCIATED PNEUMONIA

For the purposes of this article, VAP is defined according to the Centers for Disease Control and Prevention (CDC) definition for infants less than 1 year of age.[52] A meta-analysis of internationally published studies between 2002 and 2013 indicated that the incidence of VAP may range between 8.1% and 57.1% in NICU patients.[53] Risk factors for VAP are noted in **Box 4**.[54,55]

Infants who have had a diagnosis of any form of sepsis have been shown to be at risk of a worse neurodevelopmental outcome,[56] and VAP is further associated with increased morbidity, longer duration of mechanical ventilation, and longer hospital stay.[55] Infants who have a VAP may present with decreased tolerance for enteral feeds (requiring venous access for parenteral nutrition), increased apnea and bradycardia episodes (requiring increased respiratory support), lethargy (making them less able to interact with their parents), temperature instability, and increased volumes and purulence of respiratory secretion (requiring more frequent episodes of noxious endotracheal tube and oral suctioning). Nurses often play a key role in the identification of what may initially be subtle signs of an infant who is developing a VAP or other infection. Clear communication and consultation with the medical/neonatal nurse practitioner/respiratory therapy team members are necessary to allow prompt investigation and appropriate treatment. The parents should be kept fully informed

---

Box 4
Risk factors for ventilator-associated pneumonia

- Prematurity
- Low birth weight
- Length of stay
- Days of mechanical ventilation
- Endotracheal suctioning
- Reintubation
- Bronchopulmonary dysplasia
- Steroid use
- Parenteral nutrition
- Enteral feeds
- Transfusion

Of note, many of these are unmodifiable risk factors. Careful attention must be focused on prevention strategies.

---

regarding the staff's concerns, investigations, test results, and the plan for treatment. If the infant becomes too unstable to be safely held skin to skin, the parents should still be encouraged to provide comfort and containment measures.

The appropriate duration of antibiotic therapy for VAP in infants is not well defined. Therapy is typically based on the clinical course and radiologic findings, as well as the nosocomial flora and resistance patterns of the local NICU environment. However, regardless of the antibiotic used, intravenous access is likely to be required for at least several days of treatment, with the concomitant risks and discomforts that vascular access entails.

The most effective means to prevent neonatal VAP is to avoid intubation and the use of mechanical ventilation. However, until the infant is able to be adequately supported using noninvasive ventilatory modes, a comprehensive infection prevention approach may help to lessen the risk for VAP (**Table 2**).

All VAP cases should be treated as sentinel events, with review by a multidisciplinary team that strives to identify practices or processes that may have contributed to the VAP. The focus of such a review should be on opportunities for education, process, and practice change on a systematic level, not on individual performance. Each discipline involved in the infant's care may bring a different perspective to a sentinel event review. In this fashion, a multidisciplinary team approach often provides the most thorough and enlightening review.

OXYGEN SATURATION MANAGEMENT

Oxygen is a drug. As such, it should be managed with same diligence as other drugs.[57] Excessive oxygen administration is linked with both retinopathy of prematurity and bronchopulmonary dysplasia.[29,58,59] Although several large, multicenter studies have attempted to define best targets for oxygen saturation values in neonates, definitive limits have been elusive. For example, the SUPPORT trial[60] randomized extremely preterm infants (born at 24 0/7 to 27 6/7 weeks) to target saturation ranges of 85% to 89% or 91% to 95%. Retinopathy of prematurity for the survivors was reduced in the lower saturation target group but was also associated with a higher rate of mortality.

Table 2
Recommendations to prevent VAP

Hand Hygiene	Most Important for Reduction of all Infections
Wear gloves when at risk of contact with secretions	Universal precautions
Continuous assessment for extubation readiness	Discuss at least daily in rounds
Prevent unplanned extubation	Reintubation is associated with VAP
Use positioning to drain condensates away from infant	Respiratory tubing below the level of the baby Preferentially position in lateral position Elevate head of bed to 30°
Ventilator circuits changes	When visibly soiled As local auditing/policy recommends
Oral hygiene	Consider use of colostrum for oral care/oral immune therapy
Prevent reflux/regurgitation	Manage pace of enteral feeds delivery
Closed suction system	Limits atelectasis during suctioning Remains closed to potential infective agents Careful observation of secretion volume/consistency and reporting of same for team consideration
Separate suction equipment for oral and ETT purposes	Always suction the oropharynx first Suction oropharynx before repositioning infant or manipulating (adjusting/removing) ETT
Suctioning is a 2-person procedure	Person 1 monitors infant and maintains ETT position and person 2 performs suctioning 2 persons present until baby is fully resettled following procedure Monitor need for increased/decreased support following suctioning Careful titration of oxygen as needed Provide comfort and help to settle the baby Once the suctioning procedure is complete, the second person can/should be the parent

Abbreviation: ETT, endotracheal tube.
Adapted from Garland JS. Ventilator-associated pneumonia in neonates: an update. Neoreviews 2014;15(6):e225–35; with permission.

There remains uncertainty as to what oxygen saturation should be targeted. Knowing that neither hyperoxia nor hypoxia are desirable, it seems most prudent to focus care on minimizing saturation fluctuations, while maintaining targets at 90% to 95%.[8]

Based on local NICU policies, nurses carefully titrate oxygen in a continuous balancing act to maintain oxygen saturation values within prescribed targets. This process is time consuming and requires attention to detail. Hagadorn and colleagues[61] describe the variability of saturation target achievement among different NICUs, among infants within an NICU, and even for individual infants over time. Use of histograms or other trending techniques may provide insight into how successfully an individual infant is being maintained within target saturation ranges over time. An infant who is frequently below target may require increased respiratory support, optimization of caffeine dose,[8] review of feeding regime for reflux, additional containment, nursing attention, or ventilatory optimization strategies. Nurse/patient ratio has been shown to be a significant modifiable factor affecting the precision of oxygen management in the NICU.[62]

POSITIONING

Positioning plays an important role in pulmonary function for neonates. Historically, many neonatal positioning protocols were based on studies that reported the upper-most lung as preferentially ventilated.[63] Newer research has compared different body positioning for ventilation distribution in preterm infants and found that gravity has little effect on ventilation distribution. Hough and colleagues[64] identified that ventilation distribution in preterm infants follows an anatomic pattern and is not gravity dependent. There is mounting evidence that prone positioning enhances the contribution of the rib cage to tidal volume, improves thoracoabdominal synchrony, improves oxygenation, reduces apnea, reduces stress, and promotes sleep.[65–67] For practical and developmental reasons, the prone position cannot be the sole positioning strategy used. In addition, there is no evidence that any specific body position produces any long-term, clinically relevant benefits.[68] At this time, it is most appropriate to use positioning strategies that allow time to be spent in lateral, supine, and prone positions with careful observation for stress responses such as agitation, brow furrow, or desaturations. Care plans should be individualized based on infant preference and tolerance to determine which will be the most appropriate.

SEDATION AND ANALGESIA

Before the 1980s, neonatal pain was poorly understood and often underestimated.[69] Untreated pain has negative consequences on long-term neurologic development.[70] Although mechanical ventilation has commonly been considered to be a stressful experience for neonates,[71] without self-report, pain assessment and evaluation of analgesia efficacy has been challenging in ventilated neonates. Clinical trials in preterm infants using various pharmacologic sedative or analgesic therapies have raised concerns regarding safety and efficacy such that no agents are currently recommended for routine use.[71]

In light of compelling information regarding the potential for harm secondary to pharmaceutical use, nursing has embraced nonpharmacologic alternatives, which include skin-to-skin care, facilitated tucking, swaddling, minimal handling, clustered care, nonnutritive sucking, and oral sucrose. Careful assessment for other causes of discomfort is paramount. Early feeds may minimize hunger and nausea, early skin-to-skin interaction is physiologically stabilizing, and more protected rest and sleep periods allow protected healing time. Neonatal ventilation modes, such as assist control and volume guarantee, have been refined with the goal of increased comfort.

When analgesic is judged to be clinically appropriate, each NICU must have a standard of care to quantify and qualify discomfort and pain with a scoring tool, such as the Premature Infant Pain Profile,[72] resulting in appropriate use and weaning of medications. There is currently no evidence to support the routine use of sedation.[5]

EXTUBATION

Successful extubation from mechanical ventilation is a collaborative activity in which nurses play a central role.[73] The ability to provide protected time for recovery and adaptation preceding and following extubation is associated with a greater likelihood of extubation success. Practically, this means that stressful activities such as suctioning, diaper changes, physical assessment, and application of the continuous positive airway pressure apparatus will be performed well in advance of the procedure to allow for at least 1 hour of rest and recovery before and following the extubation procedure. Assisting infants to be in best possible state before extubation may provide the best chance for success. This assistance also potentially includes strategies of containment, facilitated tucking, and prone positioning to reduce stress and improve lung function.[65] A team that engages the parent to provide stress reduction strategies such as containment may contribute to a more stable respiratory system and ultimate extubation success.

OTHER SUPPORTS FOR NEONATES

The NICU is not a neurodevelopmentally friendly environment. Virtually constant stressors (painful procedures, infection, uncomfortable care regimes, light, noise, maternal separation, and sleep deprivation) all contribute to a near-constant state of stress. Such high stress in early life has been linked to both neurodevelopmental deficits and to chronic metabolic disorders such as obesity and diabetes.[74] Although high-technology interventions may be necessary to save infants' lives and physical health, nurses, other members of the health care team, and parents can have a significant impact ameliorating negative effects.

PARENTAL INVOLVEMENT

Historically, the role of parents in the NICU was very much that of spectators. Although it was generally accepted that breastmilk is a preferred substrate for neonates, and that cuddling made parents happy, the overall culture of the unit was to truly involve parents in their infants' care only as they came close to discharge home, often weeks or months after birth. However, there has been a major shift in the understanding of the importance of embedding parental involvement in virtually every moment of the neonate's life in the NICU. The science surrounding practices such as skin-to-skin care, exclusive human milk feedings, and their significant effects on early neurodevelopment is now advancing from being considered nice to do to being recognized as making a significant difference in the short-term and long-term outcome of NICU infants. Parental engagement can begin even before the birth of their infant. Antenatal consults/conversations should ideally include education about the known benefits of mother's own milk, the importance of early-and-often skin-to-skin care, and parents' unique and vital role as part of the care team. Parents should be aware that they will be encouraged to do much more than sit by the incubator and watch their infant grow.

Although the antenatal discussion may be important to set the stage for parental expectations (and presuming such a discussion has occurred), it is typically the bedside nurse who is the most integrally involved in teaching parents what they need to learn to fully engage as part of their infant's care team. Throughout such teaching, emphasis may be placed on the specialized role parents play. Only the mother can supply the colostrum and breastmilk that is uniquely matched to her infant; only the parents may provide skin-to-skin care; and, as the most constant presence in their infant's life, parents can become an important source of information to assist the rest of the NICU team to make the best decisions possible. Nurses should advocate for parents to become actively engaged in their infant's care plan, participating in daily rounds, and guiding staff on the infant's preferences, providing containment and other therapeutic measures such as comforting touch during painful procedures. In turn, as nurses develop a trust relationship with the parents, they are often ideally situated to identify when parents may benefit from further involvement with other disciplines, such as social work, psychology, lactation consultants, or other subspecialists. Having an infant fragile/sick enough to require mechanical ventilation is an extremely stressful time for parents and family. Nurses can play a key role in helping the parents to understand how they may be actively involved in their infant's care and why it is so important to their infant that they do.

SKIN TO SKIN

One of the most powerful practices known to promote a healthier infant state is skin-to-skin care.[75] The benefits of this practice have been known for many years, with identified improvements in physiologic stability, sleep patterns, pain management, stress reduction, maternal breastmilk production, nosocomial infection reduction, and enhanced parent-infant bonding, just to name a few.[76,77] "Positive or satiate early life experience, such as skin to skin contact between the mother and her high-risk infant as well as other strategies for pain and stress management, has shown beneficial effects on reducing infants' stressful responses and improving brain maturation and neurodevelopmental outcomes."[74]

Mechanical ventilation is not a contraindication to skin-to-skin care (American Academy of Pediatrics [AAP]). Of course some infants will be too fragile to move, or some supportive equipment may be unable to be safely managed or secured. The AAP clinical report suggests that 26 weeks may be the lowest gestational age to receive skin-to-skin care. In our NICU, even the most premature infants may participate in skin-to-skin care when they are deemed to be at no risk of an intraventricular hemorrhage. Clinically, this translates into very low birth weight infants waiting for at least 72 hours to participate in skin-to-skin care. Given the importance of this practice in lessening the negative impacts of the NICU environment, it can also be argued that an infant who is ill enough to require mechanical ventilation is one who could benefit the most from the practice. Moving an infant safely from a warmer or incubator to the parent's chest does require a coordinated team effort (**Table 3**). Although a standing transfer has been noted to work well in our NICUs, the transfer may also be accomplished safely when the parent is already seated in the chair.[78] The parents and multidisciplinary team work together to have a calm, quiet, and safe experience every time. Noise is kept to a minimum; lighting is dim; and although parents are encouraged to record the moment with photographs, flash photography is forbidden. The parent is equipped with a hand mirror to facilitate visualization of the infant's face.

The series of images in **Table 3** show the steps involved in transitioning a mechanically ventilated neonate out of the incubator for a skin-to-skin session.

For more than a decade at our local level 3 NICUs, the authors have safely and successfully facilitated skin-to-skin care for mechanically ventilated neonates. The nurses, respiratory therapists, and parents identify the standing parent transfer technique as the easiest to accomplish safely. This technique requires a parent who is physically able to participate in the transfer.

- Skin-to-skin duration is targeted for a minimum of 1 hour if tolerated.
  - In preparation, the parent is asked to be prepared to sit in 1 place for at least 1 hour.
- The skin-to-skin experience is typically prearranged between the parent and multidisciplinary team to ensure that the timing is appropriate for the infant regarding any planned activities or interventions.
  - An appropriate chair is brought to the bedside. It should recline and have a footrest available. The chair is cleaned by the parent before use.
  - Behind a closed curtain, the parent removes all garments from the upper body. The parent wears an adult patient gown with the opening to the front to ensure privacy.

Table 3
How to facilitate a transfer for skin-to-skin care: mechanically ventilated neonates

Roles and Responsibilities	Parent	RN1	RN2	RRT1	RRT2
	—	Assess for physiologic stability	—	—	—
	—	Consider need for ETT suctioning	—	—	—

(continued on next page)

Table 3
(continued)

Roles and Responsibilities	Parent	RN1	RN2	RRT1	RRT2
	—	Adjust height of infant warmer so that parent can easily reach infant	—	—	—
	—	Make certain all equipment reaches the chair	—	Make certain all respiratory equipment reaches the chair Maintains security of ETT	—
	The parent stands beside the infant's open bed		Maneuvers the chair so that it is positioned behind the parent	Maintains security of ETT	—

Parent leans forward, bending at the waist, and slowly lifts the infant (in the blanket or nest) to rest against chest. The infant is prone	Manages security of IV lines and infant monitoring equipment. Supports parent during transfer to arms	Prepared to move the chair directly behind the parent and lock the wheels if applicable	Maintain security of ETT. There is no ventilator circuit disconnection (maintains FRC)	Manage ventilator circuit during transfer
Parent sits down, holding infant securely	The infant's back is covered with a prewarmed blanket. Parent reclines, continuing to manage security of IV lines and monitoring equipment	Facilitates reclining of the chair and footrest into position, ensuring parent is comfortable	Maintain security of ETT	Be ready to move the ventilator closer to the parent as needed. Oxygen adjustment as required
—	Secures the IV tubing to the parent. Secures the monitoring equipment to the parent	—	Maintain security of ETT	Using medical tape, secures the ventilator tubing to the parent's shoulder and the chair
—	Documents	—	Documents	—

Note: returning the neonate to the bed, procedural steps are done in reverse. Exclusions: a suboptimal (low-lying) umbilical venous catheter, inotropes, physiologic instability, chest tube, peripheral arterial line.

Abbreviations: IV, intravenous; RN, registered nurse; RRT, registered respiratory therapist.

- All team members and parents perform hand hygiene before touching any equipment or the neonate.
- The infant wears only a diaper and is lying on a prewarmed blanket.
- The registered nurse remains present with the parent and infant throughout the skin-to-skin experience, monitoring temperature every 15 to 30 minutes, and other signs of physiologic stability.
- The registered respiratory therapist remains at the bedside until the ventilatory settings are deemed to be stable and oxygenation has stabilized.

Although skin-to-skin time should be planned to be a time for rest, with a little ingenuity and creativity, nursing staff can often perform required procedures such as limited examinations or heel sticks while the infant is being held, thus reducing the noxious effects of such negative stimuli.

Recent research has further focused on the importance of skin-to-skin care in promoting a healthy neonatal microbiome.[74,79] "Breastfed infants can gain additional [nonpathogenic] microbiota (along with those transmitted via the vaginal tract) through milk and contact with the mother's skin."[74]

SUMMARY

Care of infants supported with mechanical ventilation is complex, time intensive, and requires constant vigilance by an expertly prepared health care team. Current evidence must guide nursing practice regarding ventilated neonates. This article highlights the importance of common language to establish a shared mental model and enhance clear communication among the interprofessional team. Knowledge regarding the underpinnings of an open lung strategy and the interplay between the pathophysiology and individual infant's response to a specific ventilator strategy is most likely to result in a positive clinical outcome.

Safety is an ongoing responsibility of the entire team. Protection from untoward events such as unplanned extubation and VAPs is affected by neonatal nurse decision making.

It is increasingly evident that parental partnership is essential for positive neonatal outcomes. Skin-to-skin care, breast milk and breast feeding, and an emphasis on parental engagement are family-centered care goals.

Although the focus of this article is neonatal ventilation, care of ventilated infants requires a comprehensive approach that considers neonate gestation, pathophysiology, and inter-relationships between all organ systems.

REFERENCES

1. Keszler M, Sant'Anna G. Mechanical ventilation and bronchopulmonary dysplasia. Clin Perinatol 2015;42(4):781–96.
2. Attar MA, Donn SM. Mechanisms of ventilator-induced lung injury in premature infants. Semin Neonatol 2002;7(5):353–60.
3. Miller JD, Carlo WA. Pulmonary complications of mechanical ventilation in neonates. Clin Perinatol 2008;35(1):273–81.
4. Bancalari EH, Jobe AH. The respiratory course of extremely preterm infants: a dilemma for diagnosis and terminology. J Pediatr 2012;161(4):585–8.
5. Keszler M. Update on mechanical ventilatory strategies. Neoreviews 2013;14(5): e237–51.
6. Baker CD, Alvira CM. Disrupted lung development and bronchopulmonary dysplasia: opportunities for lung repair and regeneration. Curr Opin Pediatr 2014;26(3):306–14.

7. Smith LJ, McKay KO, van Asperen PP, et al. Normal development of the lung and premature birth. Paediatr Respir Rev 2010;11(3):135–42.

8. Sweet DG, Carnielli V, Greisen G, et al. European consensus guidelines on the management of neonatal respiratory distress syndrome in preterm infants - 2013 update. Neonatology 2013;103(4):353–68.

9. Khan A, Rogers JE, Melvin P, et al. Physician and nurse nighttime communication and parents' hospital experience. Pediatrics 2015;136(5):e1249–58.

10. Wigert H, Blom MD, Bry K. Parents' experiences of communication with neonatal intensive-care unit staff: an interview study. BMC Pediatr 2014;14(1):304.

11. Lantz B, Ottosson C. Neonatal intensive care practices: perceptions of parents, professionals, and managers. Adv Neonatal Care 2014;14(3):E1–12.

12. De Rouck S, Leys M. Information needs of parents of children admitted to a neonatal intensive care unit. Patient Educ Couns 2009;76(2):159–73.

13. Jones L, Woodhouse D, Rowe J. Effective nurse parent communication: a study of parents' perceptions in the NICU environment. Patient Educ Couns 2007; 69(1–3):206–12.

14. Latour JM, Hazelzet JA, Duivenvoorden HJ, et al. Perceptions of parents, nurses, and physicians on neonatal intensive care practices. J Pediatr 2010;157(2): 215–20.e3.

15. Leonard MW, Frankel AS. Role of effective teamwork and communication in delivering safe, high-quality care. Mt Sinai J Med 2011;78(6):820–6.

16. Miller K, Riley W, Davis S. Identifying key nursing and team behaviours to achieve high reliability. J Nurs Manag 2009;17(2):247–55.

17. Salas E, Frush K. Improving patient safety through teamwork and team training. Oxford (United Kingdom): Oxford University Press; 2012.

18. Chatburn RL, El Khatib M, Mireles-Cabodevila E. A taxonomy for mechanical ventilation: 10 fundamental maxims. Respir Care 2014;59(11):1747–63.

19. Keszler M. INSURE, infant flow, positive pressure and volume guarantee — Tell us what is best: selection of respiratory support modalities in the NICU. Early Hum Dev 2009;85(10):S53–6.

20. Harding R, Hooper SB. Regulation of lung expansion and lung growth before birth. J Appl Physiol 1996;81(1):209–24.

21. Davis RP, Mychaliska GB. Neonatal pulmonary physiology. Semin Pediatr Surg 2013;22(4):179–84.

22. Colin AA, McEvoy C, Castile RG. Respiratory morbidity and lung function in preterm infants of 32 to 36 weeks' gestational age. Pediatrics 2010;126(1):115–28.

23. Stocks J, Hislop A, Sonnappa S. Early lung development: lifelong effect on respiratory health and disease. Lancet Respir Med 2013;1(9):728–42.

24. Kasprian G, Balassy C, Brugger PC, et al. MRI of normal and pathological fetal lung development. Eur J Radiol 2006;57(2):261–70.

25. Hooper SB, Harding R. Fetal lung liquid: a major determinant of the growth and functional development of the fetal lung. Clin Exp Pharmacol Physiol 1995;22(4): 235–41.

26. Bolton CE, Bush A, Hurst JR, et al. Lung consequences in adults born prematurely. Thorax 2015;70(6):574–80.

27. Hooper SB, te Pas AB, Lewis RA, et al. Establishing functional residual capacity at birth. Neoreviews 2010;11(9):e474–83.

28. te Pas AB, Davis PG, Hooper SB, et al. From liquid to air: breathing after birth. J Pediatr 2008;152(5):607–11.

29. Bancalari E, Claure N. Control of oxygenation during mechanical ventilation in the premature infant. Clin Perinatol 2012;39(3):563–72.

30. Gupta S, Sinha SK. Newer modalities of mechanical ventilation in the extremely premature infant. Paediatrics Child Health 2007;17(2):37–42.
31. Mallya P, Gupta S. Overview of assisted ventilation in the newborn. Paediatrics Child Health 2014;24(1):1–6.
32. Björklund LJ, Ingimarsson J, Curstedt T, et al. Manual ventilation with a few large breaths at birth compromises the therapeutic effect of subsequent surfactant replacement in immature lambs. Pediatr Res 1997;42(3):348–55.
33. Morley CJ. Volume-limited and volume-targeted ventilation. Clin Perinatol 2012; 39(3):513–23.
34. Tingay DG, Mills JF, Morley CJ, et al. Indicators of optimal lung volume during high-frequency oscillatory ventilation in infants. Crit Care Med 2013;41(1):232–9.
35. Petty J. Understanding neonatal ventilation: strategies for decision making in the NICU. Neonatal Netw 2013;32(4):246–61.
36. Brown MK, DiBlasi RM. Mechanical ventilation of the premature neonate. Respir Care 2011;56(9):1298–313.
37. Miller JD, Carol WA. Permissive hypercapnia in neonates. Neoreviews 2007;8(8): e345–52.
38. Sant'Anna GM, Keszler M. Developing a neonatal unit ventilation protocol for the preterm baby. Early Hum Dev 2012;88(12):925–9.
39. Ryu J, Haddad G, Carlo WA. Clinical effectiveness and safety of permissive hypercapnia. Clin Perinatol 2012;39(3):603–12.
40. Kaiser JR, Gauss CH, Pont MM, et al. Hypercapnia during the first 3 days of life is associated with severe intraventricular hemorrhage in very low birth weight infants. J Perinatol 2006;26(5):279–85.
41. Trevisanuto D, Doglioni N, Zanardo V. The management of endotracheal tubes and nasal cannulae: the role of nurses. Early Hum Dev 2009;85(10):S85–7.
42. Wyllie JP. Neonatal endotracheal intubation. Arch Dis Child Educ Pract Ed 2008; 93(2):44–9.
43. Corff K, Seideman R, Venkataraman P, et al. Facilitated tucking: a nonpharmacologic comfort measure for pain in preterm infants. J Obstet Gynecol Neonatal Nurs 1995;24:143–7.
44. Anand KJ. International evidence-based group for neonatal pain: consensus statement for the prevention and management of pain in the newborn. Arch Pediatr Adolesc Med 2001;155:173–80.
45. Giaccone A, Jensen E, Davis P, et al. Definitions of extubation success in very premature infants: a systematic review. Arch Dis Child Fetal Neonatal Ed 2014; 99(2):F124–7.
46. Rubio-Gurung S, Putet G, Touzet S, et al. In situ simulation training for neonatal resuscitation: an RCT. Pediatrics 2014;134(3):e790–7.
47. Merkel L, Beers K, Lewis MM, et al. Reducing unplanned extubations in the NICU. Pediatrics 2014;133(5):e1367–72.
48. Gardner D, Shirland L. Evidence-based guideline for suctioning the intubated neonate and infant. Neonatal Netw 2009;28(5):281–302.
49. Bailey C, Kattwinkel J, Teia K, et al. Shallow versus deep endotracheal suctioning young rabbits: pathological effects on the tracheobronchial wall. Pediatrics 1988; 82:746–51.
50. Cordero L, Sananes M, Ayers LW. Comparison of a closed (Trach Care MAC) with an open endotracheal suction system in small premature infants. J Perinatol 2000;20:151–6.

51. Cone S, Pickler RH, Grap MJ, et al. Endotracheal suctioning in preterm infants using four-handed versus routine care. J Obstet Gynecol Neonatal Nurs 2013; 42(1):92–104.

52. Centers for Disease Control and Prevention. Criteria for defining nosocomial pneumonia. Available at: http://ww.cdc.gov/nhsn/PDFs/pscManual/6pscVAP current.pdf. Accessed January 4, 2016.

53. Murila F, Francis JV, Bland A, et al. Interpreting positive cultures of endotracheal aspirates: factors associated with treatment decisions in ventilated neonates: positive cultures on tracheal aspirates. J Paediatr Child Health 2011;47(10): 728–33.

54. Tan B, Zhang F, Zhang S, et al. Risk factors for ventilator-associated pneumonia in the neonatal intensive care unit: a meta-analysis of observational studies. Eur J Pediatr 2014;173:427–34.

55. Cernada M, Brugada M, Golombek S, et al. Ventilator-associated pneumonia in neonatal patients: an update. Neonatology 2014;105(2):98–107.

56. Alshaikh B, Yusuf K, Sauve R. Neurodevelopmental outcomes of very low birth weight infants with neonatal sepsis: systematic review and meta-analysis. J Perinatol 2013;33(7):558–64.

57. Hardy W. Managing desaturations in preterm infants. Adv Neonatal Care 2010; 10(6):330–1.

58. Deulofeut R, Critz A, Adams-Chapman I, et al. Avoiding hyperoxia in infants < or = 1250 g is associated with improved short- and long-term outcomes. J Perinatol 2006;26:700–5.

59. Birenbaum HJ, Dentry A, Cirelli J, et al. Reduction in the incidence of chronic lung disease in very low birth weight infants: results of a quality improvement process in a tertiary level neonatal intensive care unit. Pediatrics 2009;123:44–50.

60. SUPPORT Study Group of the Eunice Kennedy Shriver NICHD Neonatal Research Network, Carlo WA, Finer NN, et al. Target ranges of oxygen saturation in extremely preterm infants. N Engl J Med 2010;362(21):1959–69.

61. Hagadorn JL, Furey AM, Nghiem TH, et al, AVIOx Study Group. Achieved versus intended pulse oximeter saturation in infants born less than 28 weeks; gestation: the AVIOx study. Pediatrics 2006;118:1574–82.

62. Sink DW, Hope SAE, Hagadorn JI. Nurse:patient ratio and achievement of oxygen saturation goals in premature infants. Arch Dis Child Fetal Neonatal Ed 2011;96: F93–8.

63. Heaf DF, Helms P, Gordon I, et al. Postural effect on gas exchange in infants. N Engl J Med 1983;308:1505–8.

64. Hough JL, Johnston L, Brauer S, et al. Effect of body position on ventilation distribution in ventilated preterm infants. Pediatr Crit Care Med 2013;14:171–7.

65. Gouna G, Rakza T, Kuissi E, et al. Positioning effects on lung function and breathing pattern in premature newborns. J Pediatr 2013;162(6):1133–7.

66. Chang YJ, Anderson GC, Lin CH. Effects of prone and supine position on sleep state and stress responses in mechanically ventilated preterm infants during the first postnatal week. J Adv Nurs 2002;40(2):161–9.

67. Chang YJ, Anderson GC, Dowling D, et al. Decreased activity and oxygen desaturation in prone ventilated preterm infants during the first postnatal week. Heart Lung 2002;31:34–42.

68. Balaguer A, Escribano J, Roqué i Figuls M, et al. Infant position in neonates receiving mechanical ventilation. Cochrane Database Syst Rev 2013;(3): CD003668.

69. McPherson C. Sedation and analgesia in mechanically ventilated preterm neonates: continue standard of care or experiment? J Pediatr Pharmacol Ther 2012;17(4):351–64.
70. Kesavan K. Neurodevelopmental implications of neonatal pain and morphine exposure. Pediatr Ann 2015;44(11):e260–4.
71. Boyle EM, Freer Y, Wong CM, et al. Assessment of persistent pain or distress and adequacy of analgesia in preterm ventilated infants. Pain 2006;24:87–91.
72. Stevens B, Johnston CC, Petryshen P, et al. Premature infant pain profile: development and initial validation. Clin J Pain 1996;12:13–22.
73. Vandertak K. Collaborative extubation; best practice? J Neonatal Nurs 2008;14: 166–9.
74. Cong X, Henderson WA, Graf J, et al. Early life experience and gut microbiome: the brain-gut-microbiota signaling system. Adv Neonatal Care 2015;15(5):314–23.
75. Carbasse A, Kracher S, Hausser M, et al. Safety and effectiveness of skin-to-skin contact in the NICU to support neurodevelopment in vulnerable preterm infants. J Perinat Neonatal Nurs 2013;27(3):255–62.
76. Nishitani S, Miyamura T, Tagawa M, et al. The calming effect of a maternal breast milk odor on the human newborn infant. Neurosci Res 2009;63(1):66–71.
77. Sadathosseini AS, Negarandeh R, Movahedi Z. The effect of a familiar scent on the behavioral and physiological pain responses in neonates. Pain Manag Nurs 2013;14(4):e196–203.
78. Neu M, Browne J, Vojir C. The impact of two transfer techniques used during skin-to-skin care on the physiologic and behavioural responses of preterm infants. Nurs Res 2000;49(4):215–23.
79. Hartz LE, Bradshaw W, Brandon DH. Potential NICU environmental influences on the neonate's microbiome: a systematic review. Adv Neonatal Care 2015;15(5): 324–35.

Nursing Strategies for Effective Weaning of the Critically Ill Mechanically Ventilated Patient

Darian Ward, RN, MN, BN, PGCertCritCare, PGDipProfStud[a],*,
Paul Fulbrook, RN, PhD, MSc, PGDipEduc[b,c]

KEYWORDS

- Critical care • Intensive care • Mechanical ventilation • Nursing
- Spontaneous breathing trial • Weaning readiness • Weaning protocol

KEY POINTS

- Best evidence supports the use of a weaning protocol.
- Combining interventions helps to optimize readiness for weaning.
- Criteria-based assessment of readiness to wean should be performed frequently.
- Spontaneous breathing trials add sensitivity to ventilator liberation decisions.

INTRODUCTION

Although mechanical ventilation is a useful tool to control the work of breathing and optimize oxygenation in critically ill patients, complications can occur. Potential hazards are related to the presence of an artificial airway and the mechanics of ventilation itself. However, the risks imposed by mechanical ventilation can be mitigated if nurses use strategies that promote early but appropriate reduction of ventilatory support and timely extubation.

The process of transferring a patient from ventilatory support to spontaneous breathing is referred to as weaning, and is defined as the "transition of the work of breathing and control of ventilation from the ventilator to the patient, a little at a time or all at once."[1] This can be simple, difficult, or prolonged and the trajectory can be challenging for clinicians to predict.[2] Characteristics of effective weaning strategies include interventions to optimize readiness to wean, frequent assessment of

[a] Education, Training and Research, Wide Bay Hospital and Health Service, 65 Main Street, Hervey Bay, Queensland 4655, Australia; [b] Nursing Research and Practice Development Centre, The Prince Charles Hospital, Brisbane 4032, Australia; [c] School of Nursing, Midwifery and Paramedicine, Australian Catholic University, 1100 Nudgee Road, Brisbane 4014, Australia
* Corresponding author.
E-mail address: darian.ward@health.qld.gov.au

Crit Care Nurs Clin N Am 28 (2016) 499–512
http://dx.doi.org/10.1016/j.cnc.2016.07.008
ccnursing.theclinics.com

readiness to wean, strategies to augment and promote spontaneous breathing during weaning, and the use of spontaneous breathing trials (SBTs) to help identify the potential to liberate the patient from the ventilator. A good weaning protocol should cover all of these aspects. In this context, the aim of this article was to review effective strategies that align clinical decision-making with best available evidence to help nurses navigate the patient's path from ventilation to liberation from the ventilator (**Fig. 1**).

Optimization of Readiness to Wean

Weaning is a physically and cognitively demanding journey for the critically ill patient. From the nurse's perspective, the first consideration in any weaning strategy is to ensure that the patient is physically and cognitively prepared by applying treatment strategies that help the patient reach the point of readiness to wean. Many elements of care that at first glance might seem unrelated to weaning have a critical role to play in preparation of the patient. Reducing ventilation too early, for example, when the patient has very low energy reserves or is still under the influence of sedation is likely to result in failure. Thus, it is essential that critical care nurses not only identify the point at which the critically ill patient is ready to commence weaning but focus also on interventions that help the patient to get to that point of readiness. Promptly identifying this point opens the door to weaning and ultimately to liberation from the ventilator.[3,4]

The duration of ventilation and prospect of weaning success is heavily influenced by interventions managed by nurses in advance of reducing mechanical ventilation. The first step must be assessment of the underlying condition and management of the patient with the aim to achieve weaning success.[4] There are several areas in which nurses can assimilate information about the patient's status that can help determine the patient's readiness for weaning. Knowing the status of the patient helps nurses to identify what intervention is required. For example, measures of muscle weakness, such as handgrip strength and oxidative stress, are associated with difficult or prolonged weaning.[5–7] Also, the magnitude of change in brain natriuretic peptide levels as a reflection of cardiac strain may be a good predictor of weaning readiness.[6] The predictive value of measures such these emphasize that optimization of weaning readiness demands broad consideration of critical care interventions that address the patient's underlying condition and cause of respiratory failure, cardiac function and hemodynamic stability, cognitive function, and muscle condition. Because these factors are interconnected, optimization of weaning readiness requires a holistic approach, which is focused on removing obstacles to the patient's capacity to cope cognitively and physically with the transition to work of breathing and ventilation control. In this context, important areas that nurses can influence are outlined in **Table 1**. These include the use of delirium and sedation management protocols and introduction of early mobilization programs. Interventions such as these promote weaning readiness and spontaneous breathing capability through enhancing cognitive and physical function.[8–18] The nurse has a key role to play in terms of psychological preparation of the patient at all stages of the weaning process. Whenever possible, preparation should be consultative and negotiated with the patient so as to establish an agreed plan of care. Psychological support and effective communication are key to successful weaning.

Readiness to Wean

Although the assessment of some weaning readiness criteria, such as cognitive function, can be somewhat subjective,[3] there is growing acceptance that several factors have a quantifiable impact on weaning readiness and successful liberation from ventilation. Therefore, although a single intervention can impact weaning success,

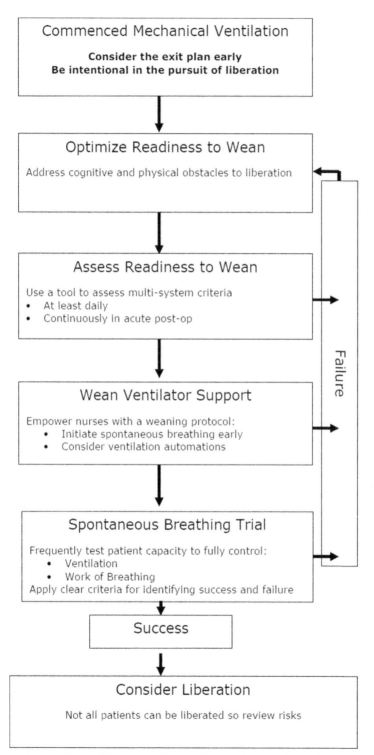

Fig. 1. Weaning a patient off mechanical ventilation. post-op, postoperative.

Table 1
Interventions influencing weaning readiness

Objective	Interventions
Enhancing cognitive function	Management protocols for • Delirium • Sedation titration Nonpharmacological interventions, such as music therapy
Enhancing physical function	Address the underlying condition and cause of respiratory failure. Cardiac function and hemodynamic stability • Fluid management protocols • Titrate medication to optimize cardiac function Muscle conditioning • Early mobilization • Airway clearance exercises • Ventilation modes augmenting spontaneous breathing
Airway management	• Noninvasive ventilation • Tracheotomy

combining several interventions together is more likely to produce better results.[19,20] Key strategies that have been shown to promote weaning readiness and shorten the duration of ventilation include the use of techniques that promote muscle strength and airway clearance, use of ventilation modes that augment spontaneous breathing effort, and early airway management decision-making, such as use of noninvasive ventilation or tracheotomy.

Weaning readiness should be assessed regularly to determine the extent to which the patient is ready to complete the transition to work of breathing and control of ventilation.[21] Frequency of assessment should be no less than daily and in acute postoperative patients should be a continuous consideration, taking into account the multisystem criteria outlined in **Table 2**.[3,22–25]

Most critically ill patients who require mechanical ventilation will present with a relatively straightforward readiness to wean picture. However, critically ill patients who

Table 2
Readiness to wean criteria

System	Assessment Criteria
Respiratory	Underlying cause of respiratory failure is resolving Adequate cough Positive end expiratory pressure 5–8 cm H_2O Pao_2 >50–60 mm Hg with Fio_2 <0.50; Pao_2/Fio_2 >150 $Paco_2$ <50 mm Hg with pH >7.25 Minute ventilation 5–10 L/min
Cardiac	Heart rate <140 Absence of arrhythmia
Hemodynamic	Minimal or low vasopressor requirement Blood pressure 90–180 systolic
Neurologic	Glasgow Coma Score >8 No or minimal anxiety Well-controlled pain Well rested; effective sleep patterns

have been ventilated for more than 72 hours benefit from a more systematic and methodical approach to differentiate between those who are ready to wean and those who have a significant risk of failure and will require further intervention to achieve readiness.[3] The Burns Wean Assessment Program (BWAP), which consists of 26 clinical factors that monitor patients' status and progress,[3] is an example of a tool designed to assess the patient's readiness to undertake an SBT with a focus on prompting optimization of factors that might otherwise compromise weaning success.[21] Use of a validated and reliable tool, such as the BWAP, reduces the risk of premature reduction of ventilatory support when the patient is unable to manage work of breathing or control ventilation.[3,26] Although not all weaning protocols may use this particular tool, they invariably incorporate consideration of similar criteria to determine when it is appropriate to progress to an SBT.[7,22–25]

The Weaning Process

Weaning is the process of assisting patients to breathe spontaneously without mechanical ventilatory support.[27] The process is incremental and it is important that ventilation parameters are changed one at a time, so that their individual effect can be observed.[28] The aim is for the patient to contribute to the work of breathing from an early stage. However, this can be very challenging for some patients who have been ventilated for several days due to muscle atrophy. Transitioning the critically ill patient from readiness to wean to liberation from mechanical ventilation in a timely and efficient manner is an essential element of critical care management, especially as prolonged weaning may increase morbidity and mortality.[29,30] Weaning techniques, such as protocols, that are used when the patient is ready to wean decrease the duration of ventilation[31,32] and may be nurse-led.[28,33]

A recent scoping review of qualitative studies highlighted that clinicians perceived weaning practices to be influenced by important issues such as interprofessional collaboration and communication, the fusion between subjective knowledge and objective clinical data, convictions about balancing individual needs with weaning systematization, and appreciation for the physical and psychological work of breathing.[34] These issues are influenced by patient, clinician, and organizational factors challenging the concept of "usual care."[35] Clinicians exhibit a propensity to favor individualized approaches to weaning[36] and there is a fine line between individualized care and unpredictable care that is not consistently tethered to an underpinning strategy or evidence. In some cases, weaning practices may be broadly similar but distinctly different from use of a protocol.[35] Without direction from a protocol, decision-making responsibility can be unclear.[37]

Weaning practices can vary substantially from patient to patient based on each clinician's knowledge, skill, and convictions. In this context, the "usual care" referred to in randomized controlled studies is an all-encompassing and at the same time profoundly ambiguous concept conveniently bundling eclectic weaning practices together on the basis they are different from the intervention under analysis. The control group in studies evaluating weaning strategies is frequently subjected to this unpredictability and variation under the description of "usual care," which can make it difficult for clinicians to make judgments about the clinical application of research.

Extubation failure and tracheostomy requirements increase with the complexity of weaning and patients with difficult and prolonged journeys have a significantly increased mortality.[29,30] This is likely a reflection of underlying disease severity and complications of mechanical ventilation.[38] Together, optimization of readiness to wean, assessment of weaning readiness criteria, and SBT performance are useful decision-making tools that support analysis and action on these issues. Routine utilization of these practices can effectively inform the clinical decision to liberate from ventilatory support. The challenge for nurses is to incorporate these activities into their usual practice for ventilated patients.

Weaning protocols

Protocols are designed to reduce the variability encountered in usual care by providing decision-making guidance.[39] The evidence for using a weaning protocol to constrain the propensity for variability in clinical practice is persuasive. Research findings favor protocols in most contexts and transcend significant heterogeneity among studies.[40,41] Recent research continues to identify that protocols led by nurses, respiratory therapists, and other health care professionals at the point of care accelerate ventilator discontinuation compared with usual care.[23–25,42] These effects can be quite pronounced in patients who are difficult to wean[23,24] and are reproducible on a large scale across multiple facilities.[25]

A recent prospective, cluster randomized controlled trial study allocated 14 tertiary teaching hospital intensive care units (ICUs) to either usual care or implementation of a weaning protocol.[25] Seven hospitals that empowered junior staff with a protocol achieved significant benefits compared with hospitals that used usual care. Reported outcomes included the following:

- Duration of mechanical ventilation was decreased from 7 to 3 days ($P = .003$)
- Time before first weaning attempt was decreased from 3.63 to 1.96 days ($P = .003$)
- Length of ICU stay was decreased from 10 to 6 days ($P = .004$)
- Length of hospital stay was decreased from 23 to 19 days ($P < .001$)
- Number of patients requiring ventilation for more than 21 days was reduced ($P = .001$)

Although these results appear clinically significant, they should be interpreted cautiously, as large statistical effects can be produced when usual care, which may be suboptimal, is used as the comparator. Usual care represents a continuum that may include broadly similar evidence-based strategies to the protocol or in other cases may deviate significantly. Thus, effect size of some protocols may be less significant or approach equivalence with usual care in departments with higher ratios of experienced clinicians.[43,44] Therefore, weaning protocols may be more effective in organizations in which there are less experienced clinicians, and their routine use should be considered as usual care.[1] Although the evidence in favor of using a weaning protocol is consistent, regardless of which protocol is used, there is a growing appreciation that other factors contribute to ventilation process and outcome variability.

Promoting spontaneous breathing

Historically, ventilation practices enforced prolonged periods of diaphragmatic inactivity that led to respiratory muscle atrophy; however, modern ventilators still induce this effect to some extent by reducing diaphragmatic work.[1,45] Recognition that diaphragmatic weakness can increase the duration of mechanical ventilation has motivated the design of ventilation modes that promote or adapt to patient effort.[46] This has been made possible with improvements in ventilator performance, particularly trigger sensitivity and flow performance, which are integral to synchronization with patient effort.[47] Once a patient is able to breathe spontaneously, strategies that promote and augment spontaneous patient effort are integral to muscle conditioning and weaning success.[5,14,20] Ventilators and ventilation modes that synchronize with and augment spontaneous effort may also contribute to improved sleep quantity and quality in critically ill patients.[48,49]

Weaning protocol automation

Although weaning protocols guide clinicians' decision-making, they often require adjustment at an individual patient level, with many possible variations. Thus, protocol-guided clinician decision-making is an example of an open-loop system. However, when clinicians deviate away from tried and tested protocols, their effectiveness may be compromised. Other factors that may influence protocol compliance are workforce skill-mix and staffing levels.[1]

Improving protocol compliance is a powerful motivator behind current trends toward the use of ventilation automation. Automated weaning protocols are described as closed-loop. Such systems involve continuous feedback of measurements of the patient's respiratory mechanics,[50] which enable frequent adaptation of ventilatory support in response to the physiologic state of the patient.[51] Automated weaning systems may support standardization of care and help to prevent errors by reducing reliance on human-based knowledge and skills to drive weaning strategies and protocol compliance.[1]

Because ventilation automation is relatively new, there is insufficient research available currently, making it difficult to compare their effectiveness in terms of weaning,[1,52] and it is difficult for clinicians to compare the relative merits of the various distinctly different closed-loop system options that are commercially available. The underpinning design principles, respiratory mechanic measurements, and use of decision-making algorithms can be quite different. Such systems include proportional assist ventilation (PAV), neurally adjusted ventilatory assistance (NAVA), SmartCare/PS, and adaptive support ventilation (ASV).[1,53] With the exception of ASV, all of these systems are essentially advanced versions of pressure support ventilation with some underpinning closed-loop automations individualizing the level of pressure support provided.[50]

In most cases, available research studies compare a single closed-loop system (eg, SmartCare/PS or ASV) to either usual care or an open-loop protocol driven by clinicians. Recent systematic review and meta-analysis indicates automations may reduce weaning and ventilation duration, as well as ICU stay, when compared with nonautomated weaning.[41,54] However, the most recent review did not find evidence of effect using automated systems other than SmartCare.[41] This may be because half of the SmartCare trials that were reviewed used usual care rather than a protocol as the control; large effect sizes have been reported when comparing SmartCare with usual care.[55] As noted previously, usual care comparisons are a convenient design that are likely to demonstrate the greatest magnitude of effect, so it is questionable whether nonprotocol control groups should be used for comparison.

When trials of ASV that used protocol-based weaning as a comparator were reviewed, equivalence or limited benefit was found.[41] Comparing automations with clinician-led open-loop protocols is a more defensible design and tends to demonstrate equivalence in terms of time to ventilator discontinuation.[56] When SmartCare was compared with clinician-led open-loop protocols, although promising effects were demonstrated, they were often less significant, approaching equivalence or in some cases favoring knowledgeable clinicians.[43,56–59] It is possible that ventilation automation may add little or no outcome benefit when compared with a well-designed weaning protocol that is complied with by knowledgeable clinicians.

Ventilation automation may prove to be most effective when it is used with patients who are not complex, especially as this is where most of the research evidence lies.

This has prompted some recommendations in favor of automation as a workload reduction strategy as opposed to clinical outcome benefit.[57] Ventilation automation may have merit if clinical workload is reduced even though clinical benefit might be equivalent or minor. Thus, it may have greater potential in resource-limited environments rather than in those with high levels of experienced staff.[1,60]

Spontaneous breathing trials

The extent to which a patient is capable of taking over control of ventilation and transition to the work of breathing demands frequent assessment.[21] This is a key decision point preceding liberation from ventilatory support. Once weaning readiness criteria have been met, and the weaning process has begun, conducting a daily SBT can help identify patients who can be successfully liberated from ventilatory support.[61] An SBT involves reduction of ventilatory support to a minimum level using low pressure support or a T-piece for a duration of between 30 minutes and 2 hours (**Box 1**). Patients who do not meet readiness to wean criteria are unlikely to benefit from an SBT.

Fortunately, most mechanically ventilated patients are simple to wean.[20,29,30] However, repeated failure of SBTs may have prognostic significance. Patients with less SBT attempts before successfully coping with the transition to minimal ventilatory support tend to have better clinical outcomes.[29,30] Although there is no conclusive evidence regarding the duration or technique of SBT,[62] the key to success is consistent use of an SBT strategy in association with regular assessment of weaning readiness criteria.

Modern mechanical ventilators often incorporate software options that include functionality to set SBT parameters and criteria for notification of the success or failure of an SBT. However, this can be confounding, as clinicians have struggled to reach consensus on the usefulness of weaning success predictors[63–65] and this may explain their propensity to favor traditional ventilatory performance predictors (**Table 3**). In general, Glasgow Coma Scale (GCS) score, respiratory rate, presence of an effective cough, and pressure support requirements are viewed to have greater utility than other more sophisticated measurements.[66] Low GCS score, hypercapnia, increased heart

---

Box 1
Components of a spontaneous breathing trial (SBT)

- Daily (or more frequent) evaluation of readiness to wean
- Daily SBT for those meeting readiness criteria
- Integrated assessment of the patient's spontaneous breathing
- Low pressure support ventilation settings 5 to 7 cm H_2O or T-piece
- Low positive end expiratory pressure (PEEP) 5 cm H_2O or T-piece
- Minimum 30-minute trial and maximum 2 hours (no evidence length increases predictive value)
- Rest patients failing an SBT for a day while reversible causes are addressed
- Propose ventilator liberation when no signs of distress in defined timeline

Data from Gupta P, Giehler K, Walters R, et al. The effect of a mechanical ventilation discontinuation protocol in patients with simple and difficult weaning: impact on clinical outcomes. Respir Care 2014;59:170–7; and Taniguchi C, Victor E, Pieri T, et al. Smart care versus respiratory physiotherapy-driven manual weaning for critically ill adult patients: a randomized controlled trial. Crit Care 2015;19:246–55.

Table 3
Spontaneous breathing trial: criteria for success and failure

System	Criteria: Success	Criteria: Failure (If Any Criterion Is Met, Discontinue SBT and Assess for Reversible Causes of Respiratory Failure)
Respiratory	• Respiratory rate <35 breaths/min • SpO_2 >90% or baseline • $Paco_2$ change <20% from baseline • No respiratory distress	Work of breathing • Respiratory rate >35 breaths/min • Accessory muscle use • Abdominal paradox • Diaphoresis Oxygenation • SpO_2 <90% Ventilation • $Paco_2$ increase of >20% from baseline
Cardiac	• Heart rate <140 beats/min • Heart rate change <20% from baseline • No arrhythmias	• Heart rate >140 beats/min • Heart rate change >20% from baseline • New arrhythmia
Hemodynamic	• Systolic blood pressure 90–180 mm Hg • Blood pressure change <20% from baseline • No or low vasopressor requirements	• Systolic blood pressure >180 mm Hg or <90 mm Hg • Blood pressure change >20% from baseline • Increasing vasopressor requirement from baseline
Neurologic	No change in mental status	Mental status deterioration • Drowsiness or somnolence • Anxiety, agitation • Decrease in Glasgow Coma Scale

Data from Refs.[23–25]

rate, and reduced handgrip strength are predictive of prolonged weaning,[5,30,67] whereas patients with reduced comorbidity and lower partial pressures of carbon dioxide tend to be weaned more successfully from prolonged ventilation.[68]

Classification of weaning complexity (**Table 4**) is retrospective and is based on the number of failed SBTs and the duration of weaning, and reflects the difficulty of predicting weaning trajectory in critically ill patients.[69] Despite meeting readiness to wean

Table 4
Weaning classification system

Classification	Indicators
Simple	• From initiation to extubation without complication on the first attempt
Difficult	• Failing initial weaning • Requiring up to 3 SBTs or • Process taking up to 1 week from first SBT
Prolonged	• Failed at least 3 SBT attempts; or • Require at least 1 week of weaning after the first SBT

Abbreviation: SBT, spontaneous breathing trial.
From Boles J, Bion J, Connors A, et al. Weaning from mechanical ventilation. Eur Respir J 2007;29:1036; with permission.

criteria, some patients will repeatedly fail SBTs and encounter difficult or prolonged weaning.[70] When a patient fails an SBT, it is essential to mitigate the risk of subsequent failures by thoroughly evaluating potential contributing factors and initiating interventions to address them. Sometimes, patients who are able to pass an SBT may lack an effective cough. In such cases, liberation from ventilation increases the risk of extubation failure and is associated with increased morbidity and mortality[71,72] and tracheostomy for airway protection is recommended.[73–75]

Ventilation Liberation

Patients should not be liberated from mechanical ventilation until demonstrating SBT success. Even when all weaning readiness and SBT criteria are met, the complexity of respiratory dynamics means liberation is still not guaranteed.[76] However, SBTs have repeatedly been identified as the most expeditious way to assess readiness to liberate from ventilatory support.[1] Ensuring optimal patient condition while promoting spontaneous breathing predict ventilation liberation success, and most patients can be extubated with minimal respiratory support, such as supplementary oxygen via a face mask. However, noninvasive ventilator support may be indicated for more complex patients; for example, those who have been ventilated for prolonged periods or have chronic respiratory disease.

SUMMARY

The risks imposed by mechanical ventilation can be mitigated by nurses' use of strategies that promote early but appropriate reduction of ventilatory support and timely liberation from mechanical ventilation. Weaning from mechanical ventilation is confounded by the multiple impacts of critical illness on the body's systems. Effective weaning strategies that combine several interventions to optimize weaning readiness and assess readiness to wean, and use a weaning protocol in association with SBTs, are likely to reduce the requirement for mechanical ventilatory support in a timely manner. In this context, ventilation automation may help to optimize weaning readiness and spontaneous breathing. Although there is substantial ongoing research into the effectiveness of weaning strategies, the science is moving rapidly, especially as mechanical ventilation equipment and techniques increase in sophistication. Therefore, weaning strategies should be reviewed and updated regularly to ensure congruence with the best available evidence.

REFERENCES

1. Branson RD. Modes to facilitate ventilator weaning. Respir Care 2012;57: 1635–48.
2. Figueroa-Casas J, Connery S, Montoya R, et al. Accuracy of early prediction of duration of mechanical ventilation by intensivists. Ann Am Thorac Soc 2014; 11(2):182–5.
3. Burns S, Fisher C, Tribble S, et al. Multifactorial clinical score and outcomes of mechanical ventilation weaning trials: burns wean assessment program. Am J Crit Care 2010;19:431–42.
4. Pan C, Qiu H. Improve survival from prolonged mechanical ventilation: beginning with first steps. J Thorac Dis 2015;7:1076–9.
5. Cottereau G, Dres M, Avenel A, et al. Handgrip strength predicts difficult weaning but not extubation failure in mechanically ventilated subjects. Respir Care 2015; 60:1097–104.

6. Farghaly S, Galai M, Hasan A, et al. Brain natriuretic peptide as a predictor of weaning from mechanical ventilation in patients with respiratory failure. Aust Crit Care 2015;28:116–21.

7. Verona C, Hackenhaar FS, Teixeira C, et al. Blood markers of oxidative stress predict weaning failure from mechanical ventilation. J Cell Mol Med 2015;19: 1253–61.

8. Schweickert W, Pohlman M, Pohlman A, et al. Early physical and occupational therapy in mechanically ventilated critically ill patients: a randomized controlled trial. Lancet 2009;373:1874–82.

9. Berti J, Tonon E, Ronchi C, et al. Manual hyperinflation combined with expiratory rib cage compression for reduction of length of ICU stay in critically ill patients on mechanical ventilation. J Bras Pneumol 2012;38:477–86.

10. Hopkins R, Suchyta M, Farrer T, et al. Improving post-intensive care unit neuropsychiatric outcomes: understanding cognitive effects of physical activity. Am J Respir Crit Care Med 2012;186:1220–8.

11. Winkelman C, Johnson K, Hejal R, et al. Examining the positive effects of exercise in intubated adults in ICU: a prospective repeated measures clinical study. Intensive Crit Care Nurs 2012;28:307–18.

12. Aghaie B, Rejeh N, Heravi-Karimooi M, et al. Effect of nature-based sound therapy on agitation and anxiety in coronary artery bypass patients during weaning of mechanical ventilation: a randomised clinical trial. Int J Nurs Stud 2014;51: 526–38.

13. Kress J, Hall J. ICU-acquired weakness and recovery from critical illness. N Engl J Med 2014;370:1626–35.

14. Elkins M, Dentice R. Inspiratory muscle training facilitates weaning from mechanical ventilation among patients in the intensive care unit: a systematic review. J Physiother 2015;61:125–34.

15. Hammash M, Moser DK, Frazier SK, et al. Heart rate variability as a predictor of cardiac dysrhythmias during weaning from mechanical ventilation. Am J Crit Care 2015;24:118–27.

16. Hetland B, Lindquist R, Chlan L. The influence of music during mechanical ventilation and weaning from mechanical ventilation: a review. Heart Lung 2015;44: 416–25.

17. Howe K, Clochesy J, Goldstein L, et al. Mechanical ventilation antioxidant trial. Am J Crit Care 2015;24:440–5.

18. Minhas M, Velasquez A, Kaul A, et al. Effect of protocolized sedation on clinical outcomes in mechanically ventilated intensive care unit patients: a systematic review and meta-analysis of randomized controlled trials. Mayo Clin Proc 2015;90: 613–23.

19. Balas M, Vasilevskis E, Olsen K, et al. Effectiveness and safety of the awakening and breathing coordination, delirium monitoring/management, and early exercise/mobility bundle. Crit Care Med 2014;42:1024–36.

20. Rose L. Strategies for weaning from mechanical ventilation: a state of the art review. Intensive Crit Care Nurs 2015;31:189–95.

21. Goldsworthy S, Graham L. Compact clinical guide to mechanical ventilation: foundations of practice for critical care nurses. New York: Springer Publishing Company; 2014.

22. MacIntyre N, Cook D, Ely E, et al. Evidence based guidelines for weaning and discontinuing ventilatory support: a collective task force. Chest 2001;120: 375S–95S.

23. Gupta P, Giehler K, Walters R, et al. The effect of a mechanical ventilation discontinuation protocol in patients with simple and difficult weaning: impact on clinical outcomes. Respir Care 2014;59:170–7.

24. Kirakli C, Ediboglu O, Naz I, et al. Effectiveness and safety of protocolized mechanical ventilation and weaning strategy of COPD patients by respiratory therapists. J Thorac Dis 2014;6:1180–6.

25. Zhu B, Li Z, Jiang L, et al. Effect of a quality improvement program on weaning from mechanical ventilation: a cluster randomized trial. Intensive Care Med 2015;41:1781–90.

26. Al-Faouri IG, AbuAlRub RF, Jumah DM. The impact of educational interventions on mechanically ventilated patients' outcomes in a Jordanian university hospital. J Clin Nurs 2013;23:2205–14.

27. Knebel A, Shekleton ME, Burns S, et al. Weaning from mechanical ventilatory support: refinement of a model. Am J Crit Care 1998;7:149–52.

28. Fulbrook P, Delaney N, Rigby J, et al. Developing a network protocol: nurse-led weaning from ventilation. Connect World Crit Care Nurs 2004;3(2):28–37.

29. Jeong B, Ko M, Nam J, et al. Differences in clinical outcomes according to weaning classifications in medical intensive care units. PLoS One 2015;10:e0122810.

30. Pu L, Zhu B, Jiang L, et al. Weaning critically ill patients from mechanical ventilation: a prospective cohort study. J Crit Care 2015;30. 862.e7–13.

31. Brochard L, Rauss A, Benito S, et al. Comparison of three methods of gradual withdrawal from ventilatory support during weaning from mechanical ventilation. Am J Respir Crit Care Med 1994;150:896–903.

32. Esteban A, Frutos F, Tobin M, et al. A comparison of four methods of weaning patients from mechanical ventilation. N Engl J Med 1995;332:345–50.

33. Lowe F, Fulbrook P, Aldridge H, et al. Weaning from ventilation: a nurse-led protocol. Connect Crit Care Nurs Eur 2001;1(4):124–33.

34. Rose L, Dainty KN, Jordan J, et al. Weaning from mechanical ventilation: a scoping review of qualitative studies. Am J Crit Care 2014;23:e54–70.

35. Blackwood B, Tume L. The implausibility of 'usual care' in an open system: sedation and weaning practices in paediatric intensive care units (PICUs) in the United Kingdom. Trial 2015;15:1–9.

36. Rose L, Fowler R, Fan E, et al. Prolonged mechanical ventilation in Canadian intensive care units: a national survey. J Crit Care 2015;30:25–31.

37. Haugdahl H, Storli S, Rose L, et al. Perceived decisional responsibility for mechanical ventilation and weaning: a Norwegian survey. Nurs Crit Care 2013;19: 18–25.

38. Esteban A, Anzueto A, Frutos F, et al. Characteristics and outcomes in adult patients receiving mechanical ventilation. A 28-day International Study. JAMA 2002; 287:345–55.

39. Ely E, Meade M, Haponik E, et al. Mechanical ventilator weaning protocols driven by non-physician health care professionals: evidence-based clinical practice guidelines. Chest 2001;120:454S–63S.

40. Blackwood B, Burns K, Cardwell C, et al. Protocolized versus non-protocolized weaning for reducing the duration of mechanical ventilation in critically ill adult patients. Cochrane Database Syst Rev 2014;(11):CD006904.

41. Rose L, Schultz M, Cardwell C, et al. Automated versus non-automated weaning for reducing the duration of mechanical ventilation for critically ill adults and children: a Cochrane systematic review and meta-analysis. Crit Care 2015;19:48.

42. Danckers M, Grosu H, Jean R, et al. Nurse-driven, protocol-directed weaning from mechanical ventilation improves clinical outcomes and is well accepted by intensive care unit physicians. J Crit Care 2013;28:433–41.

43. Rose L, Presneill J, Johnston L, et al. A randomised controlled trial of conventional versus automated weaning from mechanical ventilation using SmartCare/PS. Intensive Care Med 2008;34:1788–95.

44. Schadler D, Engel C, Elke G, et al. Automatic control of pressure support for ventilator weaning in surgical intensive care patients. Am J Respir Crit Care Med 2012;185:637–44.

45. Petrof B, Jaber S, Matecki S. Ventilator-induced diaphragmatic dysfunction. Curr Opin Crit Care 2010;16:19–25.

46. Bein T. Current concepts of augmented spontaneous breathing. New modes of effort-adapted weaning. Anaesthesist 2014;63:279–86.

47. Richard JC, Carlucci A, Breton L, et al. Bench testing of pressure support ventilation with three different generations of ventilators. Intensive Care Med 2002;28:1049–57.

48. Koldobskiy D, Diaz-Abad M, Scharf S, et al. Long-term acute care patients weaning from prolonged mechanical ventilation maintain circadian rhythm. Respir Care 2014;59:518–24.

49. Poongkunran C, Santosh J, Kannan A, et al. Clinical research study: a meta-analysis of sleep-promoting interventions during critical illness. Am J Med 2015;128:1126–37.

50. Fernandez J, Miguelena D, Mulett H, et al. Adaptive support ventilation: state of the art review. Indian J Crit Care Med 2013;17:16–22.

51. Iotti G, Polito A, Belliato M, et al. Adaptive support ventilation versus conventional ventilation for total respiratory support in acute respiratory failure. Intensive Care Med 2010;36:1371–9.

52. Morato J, Sakuma M, Ferreira J, et al. Comparison of 3 modes of automated weaning from mechanical ventilation: a bench study. J Crit Care 2012;27:741–8.

53. Lellouche F, Brochard L. Advanced closed loops during mechanical ventilation (PAV, NAVA, ASV, SmartCare). Best Pract Res Clin Anaesthesiol 2009;23:81–93.

54. Burns K, Lellouche F, Nisenbaum R, et al. Automated weaning and SBT systems versus non-automated weaning strategies for weaning time in invasively ventilated critically ill adults. Cochrane Database Syst Rev 2014;(9):CD008638.

55. Lellouche F, Mancebo J, Jolliet P, et al. A multicenter randomised trial of computer-driven protocolized weaning from mechanical ventilation. Am J Respir Crit Care Med 2006;174:894–900.

56. Burns K, Lellouche F, Lessard M, et al. Automated weaning and spontaneous breathing trials versus non-automated weaning strategies for discontinuation time in invasively ventilated postoperative patients. Cochrane Database Syst Rev 2014;(2):CD008639.

57. Inal M, Memis M, Yildirim I. Comparison of extubation times between protocolized versus automated weaning systems after major surgery in the intensive care unit. Signa Vitae 2012;7:23–7.

58. Burns K, Meade M, Lessard M, et al. Wean earlier and automatically with new technology (the WEAN Study): a multicenter, pilot randomized controlled trial. Am J Respir Crit Care Med 2013;187:1203–11.

59. Taniguchi C, Victor E, Pieri T, et al. Smart care versus respiratory physiotherapy-driven manual weaning for critically ill adult patients: a randomized controlled trial. Crit Care 2015;19:246–55.

60. Chen C, Wu C, Dai Y, et al. Effects of implementing adaptive support ventilation in a medical intensive care unit. Respir Care 2011;56:976–83.
61. Perren A, Brochard L. Managing the apparent and hidden difficulties of weaning from mechanical ventilation. Intensive Care Med 2013;39:1885–95.
62. Ladeira M, Vital F, Andriolo B, et al. Pressure support versus T-tube for weaning from mechanical ventilation in adults. Cochrane Database Syst Rev 2014;(5):CD006056.
63. Rose L, Presneill J, Johnston L, et al. Ventilation and weaning practices in Australia and New Zealand. Anaesth Intensive Care 2009;37:99–107.
64. Corbellini C, Trevisan C, Villafane J, et al. Weaning from mechanical ventilation: a cross-sectional study of reference values and the discriminative validity of aging. J Phys Ther Sci 2015;27:1945–50.
65. Cordeiro de Souza L, Guimaraes F, Lugon J. The timed inspiratory effort: a promising index of mechanical ventilation weaning for patients with neurologic or neuromuscular diseases. Respir Care 2015;60:231–8.
66. Rose L, Presneill JJ. Clinical prediction of weaning and extubation in Australian and New Zealand intensive care units. Anaesth Intensive Care 2011;39:623–9.
67. Sellares J, Ferrer M, Cano E, et al. Predictors of prolonged weaning and survival during ventilator weaning in a respiratory ICU. Intensive Care Med 2011;37:775–84.
68. Kaykov E, Vigder C, Nathan M, et al. Identifying predictors of successful weaning off prolonged mechanical ventilation among the elderly in an Israeli respiratory care facility. Int J Caring Sci 2014;7:907.
69. Boles J, Bion J, Connors A, et al. Weaning from mechanical ventilation. Eur Respir J 2007;29:1033–56.
70. Rojek-Jarmula A, Hombach R, Gierek D, et al. A single-centre seven-year experience with mechanical ventilation weaning. Anaesthesiol Intensive Ther 2015;47:204–9.
71. Huang C, Yu C. Conventional weaning parameters do not predict extubation outcome in intubated subjects requiring prolonged mechanical ventilation. Respir Care 2013;58:1307–14.
72. Hosokawa K, Nishimura M, Egi M, et al. Timing of tracheotomy in ICU patients: a systematic review of randomized controlled trials. Crit Care 2015;19:424–36.
73. Andriolo B, Andriolo R, Saconato H, et al. Early versus late tracheostomy for critically ill patients. Cochrane Database Syst Rev 2015;(1):CD007271.
74. Lim C, Ruan S, Lin F, et al. Effect of tracheostomy on weaning parameters in difficult-to-wean mechanically ventilated patients: a prospective observational study. PLoS One 2015;10:e0138294.
75. Siempos I, Ntaidou T, Filippidis F, et al. Effect of early versus late or no tracheostomy on mortality and pneumonia of critically ill patients receiving mechanical ventilation: a systematic review and meta-analysis. Lancet Respir Med 2015;3:150–8.
76. Tobin M. Extubation and the myth of "minimal ventilator settings". Am J Respir Crit Care Med 2012;185:349–50.

Special Article

Challenges in Sepsis Care
New Sepsis Definitions and Fluid Resuscitation Beyond the Central Venous Pressure

Maureen A. Seckel, RN, APRN, MSN, ACNS-BC, CCNS, CCRN[a,*],
Thomas Ahrens, PhD, RN[b,1]

KEYWORDS

- Fluid responsiveness • Sepsis • Fluid challenge • Stroke volume

KEY POINTS

- Despite many advances, sepsis remains a diagnosis with high mortality and morbidity and is the most costly condition in the United States.
- The new 2016 Sepsis-3 definitions describe patients who have higher risk for mortality. Sepsis is described as a life-threatening organ dysfunction caused by a dysregulated host response. Septic shock is a subset of sepsis in which underlying circulator and cellular metabolism abnormalities are profound enough to substantially increase mortality.
- Criteria that may be useful in identifying sepsis patients with an increased risk for mortality include the Sequential (formerly Sepsis-related) Organ Failure Assessment (SOFA) score for patients in the intensive care unit and quick SOFA or qSOFA for patients outside the intensive care unit.
- Sepsis causes physiologic changes that occur in stages, and fluids may or may not be indicated; measures that should be used to assess whether fluid is helpful or the patient is fluid responsive should be based on stroke volume changes.
- Blood pressure and central venous pressure are not reliable measures of fluid responsiveness; passive leg raise is one method for assessing fluid responsiveness and should be done in conjunctions with measuring stroke volume changes.

Because of the persistent, alarming figures for sepsis and associated mortality rates, it is urgent that dissemination of the newly released sepsis guidelines reaches the largest critical care audience possible. Seckel and Ahrens graciously agreed to an expeditious timeline in bringing this Hot Topic to Critical Care

The authors have nothing to disclose.
[a] Christiana Care Health Services, Affiliated Faculty, College of Nursing, University of Delaware, 4755 Ogletown-Stanton Road, Newark, DE 19711, USA; [b] Barnes-Jewish Hospital, St Louis, MO 63110, USA
[1] Present address: 7006 Woodbridge Creek Court, St. Louis, MO 63129.
* Corresponding author.
E-mail address: Mseckel@christianacare.org

Nursing Clinics readers to augment the pulmonary topics provided in this issue. They provide a historical perspective on the consensus work done since 1991 on sepsis definitions, criteria for early recognition, and recommendations for management. They go on to explain in detail the 2016 guidelines, along with rationale for the changes using a physiologic framework, based on the most recent evidence from three major studies. It is our hope that improved outcomes for patients will occur sooner rather than later as clinicians implement these recommended practice changes.

—Jan Foster, PhD, APRN, CNS, Consulting Editor

INTRODUCTION

Despite many improvements in sepsis care over the past 25 years, sepsis remains a diagnosis with high mortality and morbidity. Sepsis is the sixth most common reason for hospitalization in the United States.[1] One of every 23 patients in the hospital or 4.2% has a primary or secondary diagnosis of sepsis upon discharge, and sepsis is the most costly condition.[2] Patients with sepsis or septicemia are 8 times more likely to die during hospitalization (17%), have longer hospital stays, are twice as likely to be discharged to short-term care, and are 3 times likely to be discharge to long-term care than any other discharge diagnosis.[3]

Two important changes regarding sepsis care have occurred recently and are reviewed. The first is the 2016 release of the third international consensus definitions for sepsis and septic shock or Sepsis-3.[4] The new Sepsis-3 definitions and criteria are intended not only to help with earlier recognition and management but also to provide standard terminology and criteria for research, outcomes, and reporting quality measures. The terms sepsis, septicemia, and severe sepsis in the past have been used interchangeably, leading to discrepancy in reporting outcomes. It is important to have an understanding of the new information in order to incorporate the language into the everyday work with sepsis patients.

The second change involves management of fluid resuscitation and measures of volume responsiveness. It is known from the recent PROCESS, ProMISe, and ARISE studies that early goal-directed therapy did not decrease sepsis mortality versus usual care treatment protocols.[5–7] In addition, patients in the usual care treatment protocols received fewer fluids, and decreased use of central venous pressure (CVP).[5,6] A large volume of research has shown a poor relationship between CVP and fluid responsiveness, establishing that the long-term assumptions about the usefulness of CVP measures were incorrect. CVP is unreliable in most critically ill patients and is not a reliable surrogate for stroke volume (SV) or left ventricular preload and has a poor predictive value of 0.55.[8,9] CVP measures were de-emphasized in the Surviving Sepsis Campaign and Centers for Medicare and Medicaid Services Sep-1 bundle measures in 2015, and an emphasis was placed on other suggested measures of volume status and tissue perfusion assessments (**Table 1**).[10,11] Because use of the CVP is not a reliable measure of fluid responsiveness, it is crucial to have an understanding of what the research is suggesting are effective markers.

NEW SEPSIS DEFINITIONS

In 1991, the first international consensus conference to establish sepsis definitions and criteria published their findings.[12] Goals of that first consensus workgroup were to improve early bedside detection, enabling earlier therapeutic interventions along with establishing standard definitions for future research (**Table 2**). There were varying definitions and terminology in the literature at the time, which made it confusing to speak about sepsis in a common language. The consensus work also established

Table 1		
Severe sepsis and septic shock bundles		
Severe Sepsis Within 3 h of presentation	1. Measure lactate level 2. Obtain blood cultures before antibiotics 3. Administer broad spectrum or other antibiotics	
Severe Sepsis Within 6 h of presentation	4. Repeat lactate if initial lactate elevated	
Septic Shock Within 3 h of presentation	5. Administer 30 mL/kg crystalloid for hypotension or lactate $\geq$4 mmol/L	
Septic Shock Within 6 h of presentation	6. Vasopressors to maintain MAP $\geq$65 mm Hg 7. Reassess volume status and tissue perfusion by either option (licensed independent practitioner) a. Option 1: Focused Examination i. Vital signs, and ii. Cardiopulmonary examination, and iii. Capillary refill examination, and iv. Peripheral pulse examination, and v. Skin examination b. Option 2: Any 2 of the following i. CVP ii. ScvO$_2$ iii. Bedside cardiovascular ultrasound iv. PLR or fluid challenge	

Data from Surviving Sepsis Campaign Executive Committee. Updated bundles in response to new evidence. 2015. Available at: http://www.survivingsepsis.org/SiteCollectionDocuments/SSC_Bundle.pdf; and Quality Net. NQF-endorsed voluntary consensus standards for hospital care; measure set: sepsis, Sep-1. 2016. Available at: https://www.qualitynet.org/dcs/ContentServer?c=Page&pagename=QnetPublic%2FPage%2FQnetTier3&cid=1228775436944. Accessed August 1, 2016.

the concept of systemic inflammatory response syndrome or SIRS criteria to sepsis care and described the host response to infection as an activation of the immune response.[12,13] The SIRS response was defined as the presence of at least 2 of 4 criteria (see **Table 2**).

The second consensus conference met in 2001 and included 3 main goals. The first included a review of the 1992 definitions of sepsis and evaluated strengths and weaknesses. The second goal was to again improve the definitions. Finally, the third goal was to identify methodologies that improved the reliability and validity of the definitions along with ease of clinical use at the bedside.[14] Sepsis criteria were expanded beyond SIRS to include additional diagnostic criteria for sepsis (see **Table 2**). A new classification model for staging and identifying sepsis was suggested: PIRO, or predisposition, infection, response, and organ failure sepsis classification system. PIRO was modeled after the TMN system developed for cancer. Although PIRO has been shown to be a predictor for mortality, routine use of the model has had conflicting results, is challenging to use, and is no longer commonly used.[15–17]

The third consensus conference published their findings in 2016[4] (see **Table 2**). As there is no currently validated single diagnostic test for sepsis, the group focused again on definitions and criteria that could be measured clinically, be easily obtainable in all settings, provide uniformity, and reflect the current understanding of sepsis abnormality. Sepsis remains a life-threatening syndrome in which early recognition and rapid treatment are important to improve patient outcomes. The sepsis syndrome triad consists of an infection, the patient response to that infection, and the resulting organ dysfunction.

Table 2
Sepsis definitions and criteria 1992-2016

Definitions/Criteria	Sepsis 3[4]	Sepsis 2[14]	Sepsis 1[12]
Sepsis	**Definition** Life-threatening organ dysfunction caused by dysregulated host response to infection **Criteria** Acute change in total SOFA score ≥2 points baseline due to infection • Respiratory: Pao_2/Fio_2 • Coagulation: Platelets • Liver: Bilirubin • Cardiovascular: MAP, Dobutamine, Dopamine, Norepinephrine, or Epinephrine use • Central nervous system: Glasgow Coma Score • Renal: Creatinine, urine output Non-ICU qSOFA score ≥2 points: • Respiratory rate ≥22 breaths/min • Altered mentation • Systolic blood pressure ≤100 mm Hg	**Definition** Unchanged **Criteria** Documented or suspected infection and some of the following: General • Temperature >38.3°C or <36°C • Heart rate >90 bpm • Tachypnea >30 breaths/min • Altered mental status • Significant edema or positive fluid balance • Hyperglycemia Inflammatory • White blood cell count (WBC) >12,000 cell/mm^3, <4000 cells/mm^3, or >10% immature bands • C-reactive protein >2 SD above normal • Procalcitonin >2 SD above normal Hemodynamic • Systolic blood pressure (SBP) <90 mm Hg, MAP <70 mm Hg, or SBP decrease >40 mm Hg • SvO_2 >70% • CI >3.5 L min Organ dysfunction • Pao_2/Fio_2 <300 • Urine output <0.5 mL kg • Creatinine increase >0.5 mg/dL • Coagulation abnormalities • Ileus • Thrombocytopenia • Hyperbilirubinemia Tissue perfusion • Hyperlactatemia >3 mmol/L • Decreased capillary refill or mottling	**Definition** Systemic response to the presence of infection with ≥ SIRS **Criteria** ≥2 or more of the following: • Temperature >38°C or <36°C • Heart rate >90 bpm • Respiratory rate >20 breaths/min or $Paco_2$ <32 mm Hg WBC >12,000 cell/mm^3, <4000 cells/mm^3, or >10% immature bands

	Definition	Definition	Definition
Severe sepsis	Term severe sepsis deleted	Unchanged	Sepsis with organ dysfunction, hypoperfusion, or hypotension. Hypoperfusion and perfusion abnormalities may include but are not limited to lactic acidosis, oliguria, or an acute alternation in mental status
Septic shock	**Definition** New sepsis with which underlying circulatory and cellular/metabolic abnormalities are profound enough to substantially increase mortality **Criteria** New sepsis with persisting hypotension requiring vasopressors to maintain MAP ≥65 mm Hg and having a serum lactate level >2 mmol/L despite adequate fluid resuscitation	Unchanged	Sepsis with hypotension, despite adequate fluid resuscitation along with the presence of perfusion abnormalities that may include, but are not limited to, lactic acidosis, oliguria, or an acute alternation in mental status. Patients who are on inotropic or vasopressor agents may not be hypotensive at the time the perfusion abnormalities are measured

Data from Refs.[4,12,14]

Sepsis is described as a *life-threatening organ dysfunction caused by a dysregulated host response.*[4] The recognition of sepsis should include increased assessment and intervention due to the increased mortality, which is greater than 10% with sepsis-associated organ dysfunction. The definition incorporates the newer understanding of host response in sepsis in which the infection triggers both a proinflammatory and an anti-inflammatory response.[18] Patient, or host response, depends on the infection itself along with the patient characteristics of genetics and comorbidities. As organ dysfunction has now been incorporated into the definition of sepsis, the terminology of severe sepsis is no longer needed and has been excluded from the new definitions.

Since 1992, the presence of 2 or more SIRS criteria has been used to identify patients with sepsis and to describe an inflammatory response to that infection.[12] However, SIRS criteria do not describe or identify organ dysfunction and is known to be nonspecific to sepsis and present in many hospitalized patients with or without infection.[14,19] In addition, a recent study also showed that SIRS criteria have a limited sensitivity in sepsis specifically with sepsis-related organ dysfunction.[20]

A scoring system that currently identifies organ dysfunction is the Sequential (formerly Sepsis-related) Organ Failure Assessment (SOFA) score. This multifactor scoring system has been predominately used in critical care to grade organ dysfunction along with accounting for interventions; a change in the overall score of greater than or equal to 2 reflected a sepsis overall mortality of 10%.[21] The SOFA score requires laboratory work along with clinical measures and is not easily scored outside of an intensive care unit (ICU) setting due to the limitations of obtaining all the variables (**Table 3**). A new measure termed quick SOFA (qSOFA) was developed and retrospectively studied, has good predictive validity outside of the ICU for mortality, and was easy to administer in many settings.[22] The qSOFA score consists of 3 clinical variables: Glasgow Coma Score less than or equal to 13 or altered mental status, systolic blood pressure less than or equal to 100 mm Hg, and a respiratory rate greater than or equal to 22 breaths per minute. The qSOFA score is easily obtainable because it does not contain complex variables nor is dependent on laboratory values. A positive qSOFA score or 2 of the 3 clinical criteria present could act as screening criteria for sepsis with organ dysfunction and prompt additional assessment and earlier intervention in patients who are at higher risk. A positive qSOFA is similarly predictive of an increased mortality of 10% in nonintensive care patients.

The new definition of septic shock is a *subset of sepsis in which underlying circulator and cellular metabolism abnormalities are profound enough to substantially increase mortality.*[4,23] This definition was based on systematic review and meta-analysis, a Delphi study among the consensus group, and retrospective cohort studies using large patient data sets. Septic shock criteria are a vasopressor requirement to maintain a mean arterial pressure (MAP) greater than or equal to 65 mm Hg and a lactate measure greater than 2 mmol/L after adequate volume resuscitation.

The Surviving Sepsis Campaign has recommended education and incorporation of the new Sepsis-3 definitions.[24] The evolution of sepsis definitions and criteria, while seeking to improve earlier detection and patient outcomes, does contribute to confusion in the moment while that transition and translation of terminology takes place. Although the new definitions and criteria will continue to undergo validation and research, it is important to use the new language. This consensus in definitions will help to truly understand outcomes and what interventions are essential. Hospital sepsis teams should work with their coding and clinical teams to insert the new

Table 3

Sequential (formerly sepsis-related) organ failure assessment score

	Score				
	0	1	2	3	4
Respiration					
Pao$_2$/Fio$_2$ (P/F ratio), mm Hg	>400	≤400	≤300	≤200 with respiratory support	≤100 with respiratory support
Coagulation					
Platelets, 10^3/mm^3	>150	≤150	≤100	≤50	≤20
Liver					
Bilirubin, mg/dL	<1.2	1.2–1.9	2.0–5.9	6.0–11.9	>12
Cardiovascular	No hypotension	MAP <70	Dopamine <5 or Dobutamine (any dose)	Dopamine >5 or Epinephrine ≤0.1 or Norepinephrine ≤0.1	Dopamine >15 or Epinephrine >0.1 or Norepinephrine >0.1
Central nervous system					
Glasgow Coma Scale score	15	13–14	10–12	6–9	<6
Creatinine, mg/dL	<1.2	1.2–1.9	2.0–3.4	3.5–4.9	>5
Urine output	—	—	—	<500/24 h	<200/24 h

Adapted from Vincent JL, de Mendonca A, Cantraine F, et al. Working group on "Sepsis-Related Problems" of the European Society of Intensive Care Medicine. Use of the SOFA score to assess the incidence of organ dysfunction/failure in intensive care units: results of a multicenter, prospective study. Crit Care Med 1998;26:1794; with permission.

nomenclature into their guidelines and electronic medical records and to publish and present their data.

FLUID RESPONSIVENESS IN SEPSIS

The concept of fluid responsiveness and sepsis is an important one, considering sepsis is the leading cause of death in hospitals.[25] It is known that overresuscitation can lead to increased interstitial edema, accompanying tissue hypoxia and organ dysfunction.[26] Underresuscitation of patients in septic shock can result in tissue hypoperfusion, worsening organ dysfunction, and mortality.[8]

Ensuring that patients with sepsis have adequate tissue perfusion is critical to patient survival. However, the measurement of how much fluid a particular patient needs is not well established. This area is one area of sepsis management that desperately needs further research. However, fluid administration in sepsis patients is not as simple as is commonly practiced. Research has shown that approximately 50% of hemodynamically unstable patients are fluid responders with less than 40% of septic shock patients being responsive.[27] There are several key issues that need to be addressed when giving fluids to a patient with sepsis. A review of some of these concepts is important before actually discussing the management of the efficacy of fluids and septic patients.

Why Fluids in Sepsis Is Necessary

Fluids may be necessary in sepsis for several reasons. There will be changes in vasomotor tone as well as increased capillary permeability.[28,29] These changes create a relative hypovolemia. However, how much fluid to give in any particular stage of sepsis may not be clear or obvious from a clinical examination. Because of this ambiguity in fluid status, it is difficult to assume all patients need the same amount of fluid at any given point in the sepsis course. There is a general guideline of how much fluid to give a patient with sepsis when either organ failure is present or lactate levels are elevated.

The current guideline for giving fluids and sepsis is 30 mL/kg.[10,11,25,30] This generalized administration of fluids is designed to avoid underresuscitation. However, this recommendation clearly is not appropriate for everyone. The guideline is present due to the past history of not giving enough fluids to patients with sepsis. The research supporting this guideline is limited and controversial.[27,31] The assumption that patients with sepsis will all require this amount of fluid is likely flawed. The reason for this flaw is due to the multiphase nature of sepsis.

The Multiphase Nature of Sepsis and Fluid Resuscitation

Sepsis is not a single phase that can be treated similarly throughout the course of sepsis. For example, early phases of sepsis present much like the patient with hypovolemia. Fluid loss may be the result of increased capillary permeability in early sepsis. There is not likely an absolute loss of blood volume in sepsis, but a relative loss due to changes in both capillary permeability and vasomotor tone changes. However, in early stages of sepsis, it does appear that fluid administration is most likely to help prevent loss of perfusion to tissues.[32] Later stages of sepsis are different and may not respond as well to fluids. In order to understand if the patient will respond to the fluids at any given point in the septic process, precise measures of the influence of fluid administration is important. Unfortunately, precise measurement of the impact of fluid administration is not commonly done in clinical practice. Many clinicians rely on physical assessment to evaluate fluid need, a practice that has clear limitations.

Regardless of whether sepsis is in early or late phases, the measurement of possible hypovolemia via hemodynamics, specifically SV, is essential. Fluid therapy can only impact SV, which is how much blood is pumped with each heart contraction.[33] Because the only parameter a fluid bolus can change is SV, achieving a normal SV, for example, 50 to 100 mL, is the goal of any fluid therapy. If SV is restored, all compensatory changes will resolve. For example, if a compensatory tachycardia had been present to maintain a normal cardiac output, for example, 4 to 8 L/min, the tachycardia could also resolve with an improvement in SV (**Fig. 1**).

In the early phase of sepsis, macroparameters such as SV and cardiac output are lower than normal (**Fig. 2**).[34] It is at this point in sepsis when a lower than normal SV and cardiac output is present that a fluid bolus would have benefit. The goal is to achieve a normalized SV and cardiac output. Therefore, any fluid therapy should be evaluated as to the response of SV to a fluid bolus. Giving fluid without knowing the SV severely limits the clinician's ability to understand if the fluid bolus was effective.

However, there is another stage of sepsis that has been clearly defined as a hyperdynamic phase[35] (**Fig. 3**). In this phase, SV and cardiac output are either at normal levels or above normal levels. The hyperdynamic phase may be the result of massive vasodilation due to cytokine release.[36] Giving fluid at this stage is unlikely to improve perfusion at the tissue level because SV and cardiac output are already normal or elevated.

The hyperdynamic phase is also associated with microcapillary obstruction secondary to clot formation and cellular debris (**Fig. 4**).[37] Adding fluids is unlikely to help improve tissue perfusion when an obstruction is present. For example, if fluids cannot enter tissues due to the obstruction at the capillary level, then no amount of fluid will help.

This phase of microcapillary obstruction can be hidden if traditional parameters are used to evaluate the patient. For example, SV and cardiac output can be normal yet tissue perfusion is markedly reduced when microcapillary obstruction is present.

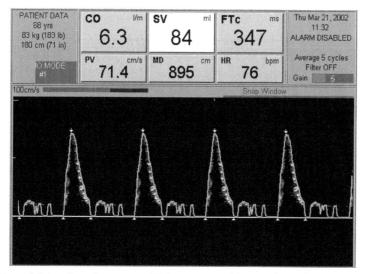

Fig. 1. Normal SV and cardiac output (CO) as measured by esophageal Doppler. HR, heart rate.

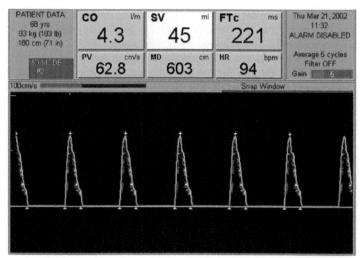

Fig. 2. Low SV and CO in a patient with pneumonia, likely in the earlier stages of sepsis.

This situation is exacerbated when clinicians use unsophisticated measurements like blood pressure or CVP.

At any stage in sepsis wherein a fluid bolus is being considered, measuring the SV is essential. Because sepsis can present to clinicians at different stages, the clinician will not know what stage is present without the measurement of SV. If SV is low and responsive to a fluid bolus, then fluid therapy is likely helpful. If SV is normal or elevated, fluid therapy is less likely to be of benefit.

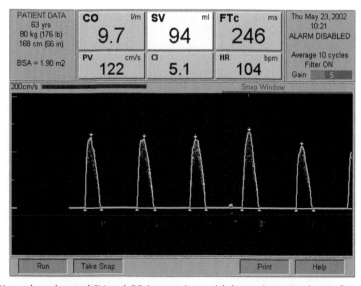

Fig. 3. Normal or elevated SV and CO in a patient with hyperdynamic phase of sepsis. BSA, body surface area.

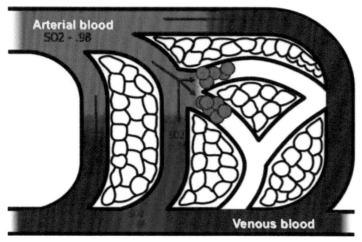

Fig. 4. Microcapillary obstruction will prevent tissue perfusion even if SV and CO are normal.

A key point to glean is that when giving fluid, the goal is to increase SV by at least 10% when the patient is hypovolemic. If SV does not increase by 10%, then it is unlikely that fluid therapy would be beneficial.

Inadequacy of Using Pressure (eg, Blood Pressure and Central Venous Pressure) to Determine Tissue Perfusion

SV is infrequently measured in patients with sepsis; this presents a problem for clinicians, who often rely on indirect indicators of volume assessment, for example, blood pressure and CVP. An MAP of 65 mm Hg is often used as a target for adequate hemodynamics.[38] In normal circumstances, elevating the MAP might improve microcirculation. However, when microcapillary obstruction is present, elevating the blood pressure cannot force fluid into the tissues. The administration of fluids may raise blood pressure but will not improve perfusion at this point. The same limitation applies to using a parameter such as CVP. Adding fluid may increase arterial blood pressure and CVP but will do nothing to improve the microcapillary obstruction. The clinician at the bedside, by monitoring the MAP or CVP, thinks that he or she is helping the patient, but in reality, no improvement in the patient has taken place because the microcapillary obstruction still exists.

Oxygenation End Points to Supplement Macrocirculation Measurement

Because of the microcapillary obstruction phase as well as the initial hypovolemic phase, fluid administration should be accompanied by a second parameter that reflects tissue perfusion. The second parameter would be an indicator of tissue oxygenation. Unfortunately, no ideal tissue oxygenation parameter exists. Probably the most helpful tissue oxygen parameter is lactate.[39] Elevated lactate levels clearly indicate a threat to tissue oxygenation in patients with sepsis. Improvement in lactate levels with fluid administration also indicates improved outcomes.[40,41] Other tissue oxygenation parameters such as mixed venous oxyhemoglobin ($ScvO_2$) or tissue oxyhemoglobin (StO_2) can provide confirmation of improvement to tissue oxygenation.[42,43] A normal $ScvO_2$ is greater than 70%, whereas a normal

StO_2 is greater than 80%.[34,44] Lower than normal values indicate a threat to tissue oxygenation. Higher than normal levels may indicate an inability of the tissues to use oxygen, for example, mitochondrial dysfunction, cell stunning, or even cell death. However, the research on these parameters has not been as clear as lactate clearance in terms of value in the septic patient. Unfortunately, all measurements have limitations. For example, lactate levels do not change rapidly. In patients with poor perfusion, lactate levels can take time to change. Real-time parameters, like $ScvO_2$ and StO_2, would be preferable. Nevertheless, $ScvO_2$ requires a central venous catheter and is a global rather than specific organ measure. StO_2 is noninvasive and attractive from that perspective, but is early in the research outcome evaluation so has not gained widespread use.

Measurement of the Effectiveness of Fluid Administration

It is important to remember that fluid administration only directly improves one parameter: SV. According to the Frank-Starling curve, as preload increases, the SV increases until the optimal preload is achieved. At the steep point of the curve, additional fluid will not increase SV and may lead to overresuscitation, potentially leading to increased ventilator days, increased ICU and hospital days, and increased mortality.[8,28] That measure that determines whether the SV is responsive to additional preload is known as volume responsiveness. Improvement in SV will lead to any other clinical change that might be measured, for example, urine output, level of consciousness, blood pressure. These parameters are all directly influenced by changes in SV. SV must be measured before fluid is given in order to determine if fluid is even necessary.

Fluid Challenge Test for Responsiveness

A fluid challenge can be performed by 2 methods: actual fluid challenges of 200 to 500 mL or passive leg raise (PLR). Both tests require measurement of SV or a surrogate of before and after.[28] The PLR test is a rapid method of predicting fluid responsiveness by using the patient's own blood volume of around 300 mL from the lower legs and splanchnic compartment and can be used in both spontaneously and mechanically ventilated patients.[45,46] The PLR mimics a fluid challenge and requires measurement before and within 30 to 60 seconds of the position change (**Fig. 5**). Acceptable methods for surrogate measurement include esophageal Doppler, transthoracic echocardiography, pulse contour analysis, and bioreactance, recognizing that there are inherent constraints due to the limitations in many of the devices.[47] As discussed previously, blood pressure and CVP are not reliable surrogates of fluid responsiveness and not recommended as a measure. Volume responsiveness is determined by the percentage change depending on the measured surrogate or greater than a 10% change if SV used.

Fluids, Inotropes, or Vasopressors?

Differentiating between the need for volume, inotropes, or vasopressors can be done by using specific hemodynamic parameters. Parameters that indicate volume may be needed include flow time and stroke volume variation (SSV). Flow time (corrected for heart rate or FTc) is an indicator of how much time is spent in systole compared with the total cycle time. A normal flow time is about 33% or 330 milliseconds. A low flow time is an indicator of possible hypovolemia.[48]

SVV is the difference between a maximal and lowest pressure wave on an arterial waveform. When the percent change between the maximal and lowest pressure points exceeds 10%, a potential hypovolemic situation is present. Unfortunately,

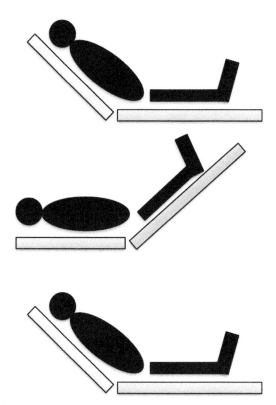

Fig. 5. PLR. (1) Obtain baseline parameter(s) with patient head of bed elevation 45° with legs flat. (2) Increase leg elevation 45° and place patient supine. (3) Obtain PLR parameters within 30 to 90 seconds. (4) Return patient to prior positioning. (5) Assess for volume responsiveness by percent change depending on the parameter (SV or other appropriate surrogates). (*Adapted from* Monnet X, Teboul J. Passive leg raising: five rules, not a drop of fluid! Crit Care 2015;19:18.)

SVV is reliable only when performed with the patient on controlled ventilation, with tidal volumes greater than 8 mL/kg, in sinus rhythm, and not having right-sided heart failure.[49] The measure may require the presence of arterial catheter or specialized monitoring equipment, which along with SVV patient limitations, restricts use to only small subsets of patients that are not typical of any ICU or emergency department. Other measures that have similar constraints to SVV use include pulse pressure variation, systolic pulse variation, and pleth variability index.[50–52]

Parameters indicating contractility or preload reduction (volume restriction) are limited, but available. For example, management of peak velocity (PV), which is an indicator how quickly blood is ejected from the baseline, may indicate the strength of the heart. The normal PV is about 50 to 120 milliseconds. A low PV indicates reduced contractility. In patients with reduced contractility, an inotrope may have value as opposed to fluids.[53]

Assessing Vascular Resistance

Parameters indicating a vasopressor may be useful are limited. Common measurements such as systemic vascular resistance (SVR) are often inaccurate and influenced by mathematical confounding. However, because of the limited ability to

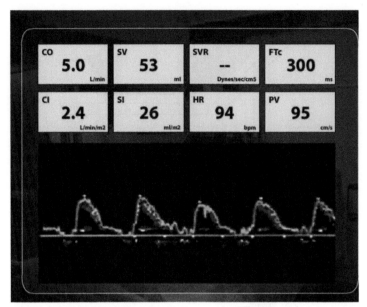

Fig. 6. Case study 1: prefluid challenge.

accurately assess vascular resistance, SVR is used to determine if pressers might be beneficial. A low SVR would indicate the possible benefits of a vasopressor in the presence of a low MAP.[54]

Case studies use parameters to determine fluid responsiveness.

Perhaps the best way to illustrate the use of parameters to assess volume responsiveness in patients with sepsis would be through clinical examples.

Case Study 1: Improvement in Stroke Volume with Fluid Bolus

A 66-year-old man was admitted to the emergency department with community-acquired pneumonia. He has the following vital signs and lactate levels, indicating the need for fluid based on the surviving sepsis campaign guidelines (**Fig. 6**, **Table 4**). Notice the SV of 53 is borderline low. In the presence of a low flow time

Table 4	
Case study 1: improvement in stroke volume with fluid bolus	
BP	90/50 (63)
P	94
RR	24
T	38.3
SpO$_2$	93 on 2 L/min nasal cannula oxygen
Lactate	4.8 mmol/L
SV	53 L/m
FTc	300 ms
PV	95 ms

Hemodynamics 08:50.
Abbreviations: BP, blood pressure; CO, cardiac output; P, pulse; RR, respiratory rate; SpO$_2$, pulse oximetry; T, temperature.

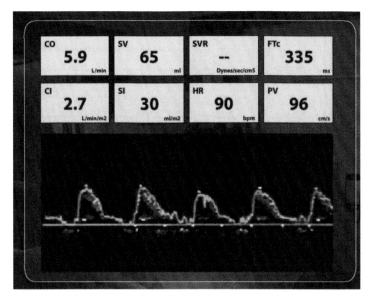

Fig. 7. Case study 1: after 1000 mL fluid challenge.

and normal PV, fluid therapy may be indicated. The only way to really determine if fluid will be valuable is to get a fluid bolus and watch for a 10% to 15% increase in SV. The patient was given a 1000-mL fluid bolus over 10 minutes. Watch for changes in SV (**Fig. 7**).

Note the SV is increased by more than 10%, which indicates the fluid bolus was beneficial. There was an improvement in the flow time as well as a slight decrease in the heart rate. At this point, another fluid bolus would be helpful. Fluid would be given until no further increase in SV was observed.

Case Example 2: Use of Stroke Volume Variation and Stroke Volume in Determining Fluid Impact

Case 2 is a 56-year-old woman who had a ruptured ovarian cyst and developed sepsis while in the hospital. On admission to the ICU, she was placed on mechanical ventilation and had an arterial line placed. She also had an esophageal Doppler placed. Note in this example that she has a low SV (33) by both measurements. In addition, she has a low flow time (257) and an increased SVV (19) (**Fig. 8**). She is also tachycardic but seems to have good contractility as indicated by a PV that is normal (103). She

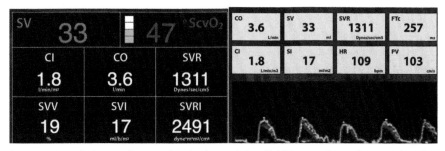

Fig. 8. Case study 2: use of SVV and SV in determining fluid impact; hemodynamics baseline.

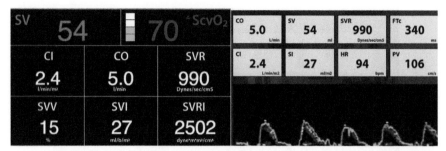

Fig. 9. Case study 2: use of SVV and SV in determining fluid impact; after initial fluid bolus.

appears to have poor tissue perfusion as indicated by the low mixed venous oxyhemo-globin level (47). Based on this information, she is a good candidate for fluid therapy. She was given 1000 mL of lactated Ringers.

After initial fluid bolus
Following the administration of fluid, notice the significant increase of more than 10% in SV along with a continued increased SVV as measured by both devices, which would indicate a need for another fluid bolus **(Fig. 9)**.

After second fluid bolus
Following the second fluid bolus, notice there was no significant change in SV as measured by either device. The SVV did improve from 15 to 12, but because this parameter is less direct of a measure of SV, no further therapy with fluids is likely indi-cated **(Fig. 10)**.

Case Study 3: Hyperdynamic Phase of Sepsis Where Fluid Therapy Is Unlikely to Be of Value

The hyperdynamic phase of sepsis with fluid therapy is unlikely to be of value **(Fig. 11)**.
Case 3 is a 62-year-old man who fell out of an automobile and suffered significant abdominal and head injuries. After 3 days in ICU, he developed sepsis. On the fifth day, he became hypotensive (BP 82/44, MAP of 57), and the question was raised "does he need fluid?".
Notice the SV is normal or slightly elevated (101). This patient is likely in the hyper-dynamic phase of sepsis. The SVV of 6% indicates hypovolemia is unlikely. He has a low SVR of 600 as well as an increased mixed venous oxyhemoglobin; based on this information, fluid therapy is unlikely to benefit this patient. A vasopressor such as norepinephrine may be beneficial.

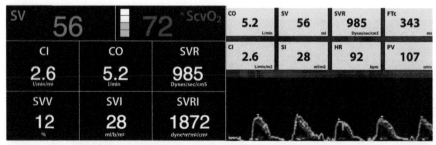

Fig. 10. Case study 2: use of SVV and SV in determining fluid impact; after second fluid bolus.

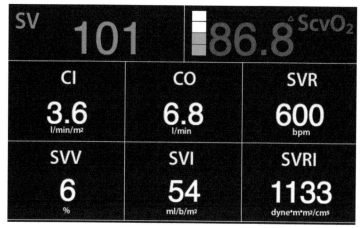

Fig. 11. Case study 3: hyperdynamic phase of sepsis where fluid therapy is unlikely to be of value; hemodynamics.

SUMMARY

Fluid administration in sepsis needs to be governed by the measurement of SV if it all possible. Giving fluid without measuring SV may lead to either overresuscitation or underresuscitation. In addition, in the hyperdynamic phase of sepsis, fluid administration may appear to be beneficial by changing parameters such as blood pressure but not really impacting improvement of tissue perfusion or oxygenation. If at all possible, measuring both flow, for example, SV, and tissue oxygenation parameter, such as lactate or mixed venous oxyhemoglobin ($ScvO_2$), is more likely to provide better information regarding the effectiveness or even the need of fluid therapy.

The understanding and treatment of sepsis have changed dramatically from the first consensus definitions in 1992 and the first sepsis guidelines in 2004. However, there is still work to do in describing and identifying sepsis patients that need early intervention and improving mortality. Interventions such as fluids should be based on evidence-based processes that are directly linked to better outcomes.

REFERENCES

1. Elixhauser A, Friedman B, Stranges E. Septicemia in U.S. hospitals. HCUP Statistical Brief #122 2011. Available at: http://www.hcup-us.ahrq.gov/reports/statbriefs/sb122.pdf. Accessed August 1, 2016.
2. Wier LM, Levit K, Stranges E, et al. HCUP facts and figures: statistics on hospital-based care in the United States, 2009. 2009. Available at: http://www.hcup-us.ahrq.gov/reports/factsandfigures/2009/pdfs/FF_report_2009.pdf. Accessed August 1, 2016.
3. Hall MJ, Williams SN, DeFrances CJ, et al. Inpatient care for septicemia or sepsis: a challenge for patients and hospitals. NCHS Date Brief 2011;62:1–8.
4. Singer M, Deutschman CS, Seymour CW, et al. The third international consensus definitions for sepsis and septic shock (Sepsis-3). JAMA 2016;315:801–10.
5. Mouncey PR, Osborn TM, Power GS, et al. Trial of early, goal-directed resuscitation for septic shock. N Engl J Med 2015;372:1301–11.
6. The ProCESS Investigators. A randomized trial of protocol-based care for early septic shock. N Engl J Med 2014;370:1683–93.

7. ARISE Investigators, ANZICS Clinical Trials Group. Goal-directed resuscitation for patients with early septic shock. N Engl J Med 2014;371:1496–506.

8. Marik PE, Monnet X, Teboul J. Hemodynamic parameters to guide fluid therapy. Ann Intensive Care 2011;1:1.

9. Marik PE, Baram M, Bahid B. Does central venous pressure predict fluid responsiveness? A systematic review of the literature and the tale of seven mares. Chest 2008;134:172–8.

10. Surviving Sepsis Campaign Executive Committee. Updated bundles in response to new evidence. 2015. Available at: http://www.survivingsepsis.org/SiteCollection Documents/SSC_Bundle.pdf. Accessed August 1, 2016.

11. Quality Net. NQF-endorsed voluntary consensus standards for hospital care; measure set: sepsis, Sep-1. 2016. Availabe at: Available at: https://www. qualitynet.org/dcs/ContentServer?c=Page&pagename=QnetPublic%2FPage% 2FQnetTier3&cid=1228775436944. Accessed August 1, 2016.

12. American College of Chest Physicians/Society of Critical Care Medicine Consensus Conference: definitions for sepsis and organ failure and guidelines for the use of innovative therapies in sepsis. Crit Care Med 1992;20:864–74.

13. Vincent JL, Martinez EO, Silva E. Evolving concepts in sepsis definition. Crit Care Nurs Clin North Am 2011;23:29–39.

14. Levy MM, Fink MP, Marshall JC, et al. 2001 SCCM/ESICM/ACCP/ATS/SIS International Sepsis Definition Conference. Intensive Care Med 2003;29:530–8. Available at: http://www.survivingsepsis.org/SiteCollectionDocuments/About-Barcelona-Declaration.pdf. Accessed August 1, 2016.

15. Opal SM. Concept of PIRO as a new conceptual framework to understand sepsis. Pediatr Crit Care Med 2005;6:S55–60.

16. Marshall JC. The PIRO (predisposition, insult, response, organ dysfunction) model: toward a staging system for acute illness. Virulence 2014;5:27–35.

17. Granja C, Povoa P, Lobo C, et al. The predisposition, infection, response and organ failure (PIRO) sepsis classification system: results of hospital mortality using a novel concept and methodological approach. PLoS One 2013;8:e53885.

18. Angus DC, van der Poll T. Severe sepsis and septic shock. N Engl J Med 2013; 369:840–51.

19. Curpek MM, Zadravecz FJ, Winslow C, et al. Incidence and prognostic value of the systemic inflammatory response syndrome and organ dysfunctions in ward patients. Am J Respir Crit Care Med 2015;192:958–64.

20. Kaurkone K, Bailey M, Pitcher, et al. Systemic inflammatory response syndrome criteria in defining severe sepsis. N Engl J Med 2015;372:1629–38.

21. Vincent JL, de Mendonca A, Cantraine F, et al. Working group on "Sepsis-Related Problems" of the European Society of intensive Care Medicine. Use of the SOFA score to assess the incidence of organ dysfunction/failure in intensive care units: results of a multicenter, prospective study. Crit Care Med 1998;26:1793–800.

22. Seymour CW, Lie VX, Iwashyna TJ, et al. Assessment of clinical criteria for sepsis for the third international consensus definitions for sepsis and sepsis shock (Sepsis-3). JAMA 2016;315:762–74.

23. Shankar-Hari M, Phillips GS, Levy ML, et al. Developing a new definition and assessing new clinical criteria for septic shock for the third international consensus definitions for sepsis and septic shock (Sepsis-3). JAMA 2016;315:775–87.

24. Surviving Sepsis Campaign. Surviving sepsis campaign responds to Sepsis-3. 2016. Available at: http://www.survivingsepsis.org/SiteCollectionDocuments/ SSC-Statements-Sepsis-Definitions-3-2016.pdf. Accessed August 1, 2016.

25. Dellinger RP, Levy MM, Rhodes A, et al. Surviving Sepsis Campaign: International Guidelines for Management of Severe Sepsis and Septic Shock. Crit Care Med 2012;2013(41):580–637.
26. Landesberg G, Gilon D, Meroz Y, et al. Diastolic dysfunction and mortality in severe sepsis and septic shock. Eur Heart J 2012;33:895–903.
27. Marik P, Bellomo R. A rationale approach to giving fluid in sepsis. Br J Anaesth 2016;116:339–49.
28. Gattinoni L, Cressoni M, Brazzi L. Fluids in ARDS: from onset through recovery. Curr Opin Crit Care 2014;20(4):373.
29. Ait-Oufella H, Maury E, Lehoux S, et al. The endothelium: physiological functions and role in microcirculatory failure during severe sepsis. Intensive Care Med 2010;36:1286–98.
30. Jones AE, Puskarich MA. The Surviving Sepsis Campaign guidelines 2012: update for emergency physicians. Ann Emerg Med 2014;63:35–47.
31. Madhusudan P, Vijayaraghavan BKT, Cove ME. Fluid resuscitation in sepsis: re-examining the paradigm. Biomed Res Int 2014;2014:984082.
32. Nguyen HB, Jaehne AK, Jayaprakash N. Early goal-directed therapy in severe sepsis and septic shock: insights and comparisons to ProCESS, ProMISe, and ARISE. Crit Care 2016;20:160.
33. Johnson A, Ahrens T. Stroke volume optimization: the new hemodynamic algorithm. Crit Care Nurse 2015;35:11–27.
34. Ahrens T. Hemodynamics in sepsis. AACN Adv Crit Care 2006;17:435–45.
35. Kanoore Edui VS, Ince C, Dubin A. What is microcirculatory shock? Curr Opin Crit Care 2015;21:245–52.
36. Ait-Qufella H, Bourcier S, Lehous S, et al. Microcirculatory disorders during septic shock. Curr Opin Crit Care 2015;21:271–5.
37. Trzeciak S, Dellinger RP, Parrillo JE, et al. Microcirculatory Alterations in Resuscitation and Shock Investigators. Early microcirculatory perfusion derangements in patients with severe sepsis and septic shock: relationship to hemodynamics, oxygen transport, and survival. Ann Emerg Med 2007;49:88–98.
38. Silva S, Teboul JL. Defining the adequate arterial pressure target during septic shock: not a 'micro' issue but the microcirculation can help. Crit Care 2011;15:1004.
39. Bakker J, Nijsten MW, Jansen TC. Clinical use of lactate monitoring in critically ill patients. Ann Intensive Care 2013;3:12.
40. Mikkelsen M, Miltiades A, Gaieski D, et al. Serum lactate is associated with mortality in severe sepsis independent of organ failure and shock. Crit Care Med 2009;37:1670–7.
41. Jansen TC, van Bommel J, Schoonderbeek FJ, et al. Early lactate-guided therapy in intensive care unit patients: a multicenter, open-label, randomized controlled trial. Am J Respir Crit Care Med 2010;182:752–61.
42. Worapratya P, Wanjaroenchaisuk A, Joraluck J, et al. Success of applying early goal-directed therapy for septic shock patients in the emergency department. Open Access Emerg Med 2016;8:1–6.
43. Samrai RS, Nicolas L. Near infrared spectroscopy (NIRS) derived tissue oxygenation in critical illness. Clin Invest Med 2015;38:E285–95.
44. Mitchell C. Tissue oxygenation monitoring as a guide for trauma resuscitation. Crit Care Nurse 2016;36:12–70.
45. Monnet X, Teboul J. Passive leg raising: five rules, not a drop of fluid! Crit Care 2015;19:18.

46. Monnet X, Teboul J. Assessment of volume responsiveness during mechanical ventilation: recent advances. Crit Care 2013;17:217.
47. Cherpanath TG, Hirsch A, Geerts BF, et al. Predicting fluid responsiveness by passive leg raising: a systematic review and meta-analysis of 23 clinical trials. Crit Care Med 2016;44:981–91.
48. Chew HC, Devanand A, Phua GC, et al. Oesophageal Doppler ultrasound in the assessment of haemodynamic status of patients admitted to the medical intensive care unit with septic shock. Ann Acad Med Singapore 2009;38:699–703.
49. Carsetti A, CeCconi M, Rhondes A. Fluid bolus therapy: monitoring and predicting fluid responsiveness. Curr Opin Crit Care 2015;21:388–94.
50. Naik BI, Durieux ME. Hemodynamic monitoring devices: putting it all together. Best Pract Res Clin Anaesthesiol 2014;28:477–88.
51. MacKenzie DC, Noble VE. Assessing volume status and fluid responsiveness in the emergency department. Clin Exp Emerg Med 2014;1:67–77.
52. McCanny P, Colreavy F, Bakker J, et al. Haemodynamic monitoring and management: skills and techniques. 2013. Available at: http://pact.esicm.org/media/HaemMon%20and%20Mgt%208%20April%202013%20final.pdf. Accessed August 1, 2016.
53. Prentice D, Sona C. Esophageal Doppler monitoring for hemodynamic assessment. Crit Care Nurs Clin North Am 2006;18:189–93.
54. Overgaard CB, Dzavik V. Inotropes and vasopressors: review of physiology and clinical use in cardiovascular disease. Circulation 2008;118:1047–56.

UNITED STATES POSTAL SERVICE® Statement of Ownership, Management, and Circulation (All Periodicals Publications Except Requester Publications)

1. Publication Title	2. Publication Number	3. Filing Date
CRITICAL CARE NURSING CLINICS OF NORTH AMERICA	006 – 273	9/18/16

4. Issue Frequency	5. Number of Issues Published Annually	6. Annual Subscription Price
MAR, JUN, SEP, DEC	4	$144.00

7. Complete Mailing Address of Known Office of Publication (Not printer) (Street, city, county, state, and ZIP+4®)

ELSEVIER INC.
360 PARK AVENUE SOUTH
NEW YORK, NY 10010-1710

Contact Person
STEPHEN R. BUSHING

Telephone (include area code)
215-239-3688

8. Complete Mailing Address of Headquarters or General Business Office of Publisher (Not printer)

ELSEVIER INC.
360 PARK AVENUE SOUTH
NEW YORK, NY 10010-1710

9. Full Names and Complete Mailing Addresses of Publisher, Editor, and Managing Editor (Do not leave blank)

Publisher (Name and complete mailing address)
ADRIANNE BRIGIDO, ELSEVIER INC.
1600 JOHN F KENNEDY BLVD. SUITE 1800
PHILADELPHIA, PA 19103-2899

Editor (Name and complete mailing address)
KERRY HOLLAND, ELSEVIER INC.
1600 JOHN F KENNEDY BLVD. SUITE 1800
PHILADELPHIA, PA 19103-2899

Managing Editor (Name and complete mailing address)
PATRICK MANLEY, ELSEVIER INC.
1600 JOHN F KENNEDY BLVD. SUITE 1800
PHILADELPHIA, PA 19103-2899

10. Owner (Do not leave blank. If the publication is owned by a corporation, give the name and address of the corporation immediately followed by the names and addresses of all stockholders owning or holding 1 percent or more of the total amount of stock. If not owned by a corporation, give the names and addresses of the individual owners. If owned by a partnership or other unincorporated firm, give its name and address as well as those of each individual owner. If the publication is published by a nonprofit organization, give its name and address.)

Full Name	Complete Mailing Address
WHOLLY OWNED SUBSIDIARY OF REED/ELSEVIER, US HOLDINGS	1600 JOHN F KENNEDY BLVD. SUITE 1800 PHILADELPHIA, PA 19103-2899

11. Known Bondholders, Mortgagees, and Other Security Holders Owning or Holding 1 Percent or More of Total Amount of Bonds, Mortgages, or Other Securities. If none, check box ▶ ☐ None

Full Name	Complete Mailing Address
N/A	

12. Tax Status (For completion by nonprofit organizations authorized to mail at nonprofit rates) (Check one)
The purpose, function, and nonprofit status of this organization and the exempt status for federal income tax purposes:
☐ Has Not Changed During Preceding 12 Months
☐ Has Changed During Preceding 12 Months (Publisher must submit explanation of change with this statement)

13. Publication Title	14. Issue Date for Circulation Data Below
CRITICAL CARE NURSING CLINICS OF NORTH AMERICA	JUNE 2016

15. Extent and Nature of Circulation		Average No. Copies Each Issue During Preceding 12 Months	No. Copies of Single Issue Published Nearest to Filing Date
a. Total Number of Copies (Net press run)		260	283
b. Paid Circulation (By Mail and Outside the Mail)	(1) Mailed Outside-County Paid Subscriptions Stated on PS Form 3541 (Include paid distribution above nominal rate, advertiser's proof copies, and exchange copies)	142	146
	(2) Mailed In-County Paid Subscriptions Stated on PS Form 3541 (Include paid distribution above nominal rate, advertiser's proof copies, and exchange copies)	0	0
	(3) Paid Distribution Outside the Mails Including Sales Through Dealers and Carriers, Street Vendors, Counter Sales, and Other Paid Distribution Outside USPS®	39	48
	(4) Paid Distribution by Other Classes of Mail Through the USPS (e.g., First-Class Mail®)	0	0
c. Total Paid Distribution [Sum of 15b (1), (2), (3), and (4)]		181	194
d. Free or Nominal Rate Distribution (By Mail and Outside the Mail)	(1) Free or Nominal Rate Outside-County Copies included on PS Form 3541	31	59
	(2) Free or Nominal Rate In-County Copies Included on PS Form 3541	0	0
	(3) Free or Nominal Rate Copies Mailed at Other Classes Through the USPS (e.g., First-Class Mail)	0	0
	(4) Free or Nominal Rate Distribution Outside the Mail (Carriers or other means)	0	0
e. Total Free or Nominal Rate Distribution (Sum of 15d (1), (2), (3) and (4))		31	59
f. Total Distribution (Sum of 15c and 15e)		212	253
g. Copies not Distributed (See instructions to Publishers #4 (page #3))		48	30
h. Total (Sum of 15f and g)		260	283
i. Percent Paid (15c divided by 15f times 100)		85%	77%

* If you are claiming electronic copies, go to line 16 on page 3. If you are not claiming electronic copies, skip to line 17 on page 3.

16. Electronic Copy Circulation	Average No. Copies Each Issue During Preceding 12 Months	No. Copies of Single Issue Published Nearest to Filing Date
a. Paid Electronic Copies	0	0
b. Total Paid Print Copies (Line 15c) + Paid Electronic Copies (Line 16a)	181	194
c. Total Print Distribution (Line 15f) + Paid Electronic Copies (Line 16a)	212	253
d. Percent Paid (Both Print & Electronic Copies) (16b divided by 16c × 100)	85%	77%

☒ I certify that 50% of all my distributed copies (electronic and print) are paid above a nominal price.

17. Publication of Statement of Ownership
☒ If the publication is a general publication, publication of this statement is required. Will be printed in the DECEMBER 2016 issue of this publication.
☐ Publication not required.

18. Signature and Title of Editor, Publisher, Business Manager, or Owner	Date
STEPHEN R. BUSHING – INVENTORY DISTRIBUTION CONTROL MANAGER	9/18/16

I certify that all information furnished on this form is true and complete. I understand that anyone who furnishes false or misleading information on this form or who omits material or information requested on the form may be subject to criminal sanctions (including fines and imprisonment) and/or civil sanctions (including civil penalties).

PS Form 3526, July 2014 (Page 1 of 4 (see instructions page 4)) PSN: 7530-01-000-9931 PRIVACY NOTICE: See our privacy policy on www.usps.com

PS Form 3526, July 2014 (Page 3 of 4)

PRIVACY NOTICE: See our privacy policy on www.usps.com

Moving?

Make sure your subscription moves with you!

To notify us of your new address, find your **Clinics Account Number** (located on your mailing label above your name), and contact customer service at:

Email: journalscustomerservice-usa@elsevier.com

800-654-2452 (subscribers in the U.S. & Canada)
314-447-8871 (subscribers outside of the U.S. & Canada)

Fax number: 314-447-8029

Elsevier Health Sciences Division
Subscription Customer Service
3251 Riverport Lane
Maryland Heights, MO 63043

*To ensure uninterrupted delivery of your subscription,
please notify us at least 4 weeks in advance of move.

ELSEVIER

Printed and bound by CPI Group (UK) Ltd, Croydon, CR0 4YY

07/10/2024

01040503-0008